Problem Solving in Child and Adolescent Psychotherapy

A Skills-Based, Collaborative Approach

KATHARINA MANASSIS

THE GUILFORD PRESS
New York   London

© 2012 The Guilford Press
A Division of Guilford Publications, Inc.
72 Spring Street, New York, NY 10012
www.guilford.com

Printed in the United States of America

This book is printed on acid-free paper.

Last digit is print number: 9 8 7 6 5 4 3 2 1

The author has checked with sources believed to be reliable in her efforts to provide information
that is complete and generally in accord with the standards of practice that are accepted at the
time of publication. However, in view of the possibility of human error or changes in behavioral,
mental health, or medical sciences, neither the author, nor the editor and publisher, nor any other
party who has been involved in the preparation or publication of this work warrants that the
information contained herein is in every respect accurate or complete, and they are not responsible
for any errors or omissions or the results obtained from the use of such information. Readers are
encouraged to confirm the information contained in this book with other sources.

Library of Congress Cataloging-in-Publication Data

Manassis, Katharina.
   Problem solving in child and adolescent psychotherapy : a skills-based, collaborative
approach / Katharina Manassis.
      p. cm.
   Includes bibliographical references and index.
   ISBN 978-1-4625-0370-4 (hardcover : alk. paper)
   1. Child psychotherapy.   2. Adolescent psychotherapy.   3. Problem solving.   I. Title.
   RJ504.M32 2012
   618.92′8914—dc23
                                                                            2011052988

*To the children, adolescents, and families
I have treated, whose courage and perseverance
in seeking to overcome their problems
are truly inspiring*

About the Author

Katharina Manassis, MD, FRCPC, is Staff Psychiatrist and Senior Associate Scientist at the Hospital for Sick Children in Toronto, where she founded and continues to work in the Anxiety Disorders Program for children and youth. The Program focuses on the development and scientific evaluation of cognitive-behavioral treatments. Dr. Manassis is also Professor in the Department of Psychiatry at the University of Toronto and a member of the Human Development and Applied Psychology Department at the Ontario Institute for Studies in Education. These appointments allow her to supervise graduate students, residents, and fellows in the treatment and study of childhood anxiety. Dr. Manassis leads several funded research studies to better understand and treat childhood anxiety disorders. She has published over 60 papers in professional journals in this field and is the author of two widely read books for parents, *Keys to Parenting Your Anxious Child* and *Helping Your Teenager Beat Depression,* as well as books for child mental health professionals on cognitive-behavioral therapy and problem solving.

Acknowledgments

I would like to thank Ms. Phyllis Earley for her formatting and administrative suggestions, Ms. Lisa Fiksenbaum for her assistance with background research, and the Department of Psychiatry, Hospital for Sick Children, for supporting me in allocating time to complete this book. Also, many thanks to the helpful editorial staff at The Guilford Press.

Contents

PROBLEM SOLVING
IN CHILD AND ADOLESCENT
PSYCHOTHERAPY

Chapter 1

What Is Problem Solving?

Mark was stuck. His college applications were due in a few days, but he couldn't decide where to apply. His father expected him to attend his own alma mater, but Mark had heard some negative comments about it and did not want to follow his father's advice. An out-of-state program interested Mark, but he wasn't sure if his family would support him in moving away from home. Mark had never left home for more than a night or two, and so he wasn't sure he could manage a big move either. Within Mark's hometown, there was another college that had a good reputation, but he didn't know much about its programs. Mark started to panic: how could he make this decision that was going to affect the rest of his life? He didn't know where to start.

Not every problem is as significant as the one Mark is facing, but many problems are difficult to solve without a clear plan. By the end of this book, you will learn how to develop a problem-solving plan and will have a good idea of how to help children and teens like Mark apply it. As a child psiatrist and psychotherapist, I have found problem solving to be one of the most useful and appreciated techniques for helping youth handle challenging situations more effectively and independently. It can be applied with children and adolescents struggling with a variety of emotional, behavioral, or academic problems. It can be learned in one-to-one therapy situations or in small groups. With a bit of thought, it can be applied with youth of diverse ages and developmental levels.

Problem solving follows certain predictable steps and therefore can be used by professionals with diverse levels of mental health training. This fact implies two things: (1) you may be able to apply the ideas in this book even if you have not had extensive training in psychology or psychotherapy; and (2) problem solving has the potential for broad use in the community, including use in primary care. Its widespread use in primary care allows problem solving to be one of the most accessible forms of psychotherapy for many children and families.

DEFINING PROBLEM SOLVING

Problem solving is a collaborative approach in which the therapist and the client work together to find and apply new solutions to a particular dilemma. It is collaborative in that the therapist is not presumed to have the "right" solution to the problem and therefore must work with the client to find solutions that are acceptable to him or her and relevant to his or her life circumstances. One assumes that there are multiple possible solutions and the best solution is determined empirically, by trying out and evaluating options until finding one that is helpful.

The focus of problem solving is addressing a particular dilemma or decision rather than changing broader patterns of thinking, feeling, or behaving. Of course, if the same solution works well in more than one situation, that solution may become habitual over time. The goal of problem solving, however, is not necessarily to form new psychological habits but rather to develop an approach to thinking about and handling challenging situations.

Problem solving is familiar to many mental health professionals as a therapeutic tool and sometimes seems almost too simple an approach to complex psychological problems. Simple approaches are not always easy to apply, though, as the examples in this book will illustrate. On the other hand, simple approaches like problem solving can sometimes offer a practical, encouraging start to addressing complex issues. For example, Mark may not be able to resolve all aspects of his relationship with his authoritarian father this week, but he can develop a logical approach to the college application dilemma this week. The confidence he gains by doing so will encourage him and may eventually contribute to a healthier relationship with his father.

WHEN CAN YOU USE PROBLEM SOLVING?

Problem solving can be used in any situation where an individual has a choice and at least some influence on the outcome but there is no clear-cut rule to follow. Children have more limited control over their environments than adults do; so, their ability to make choices and influence outcomes may be restricted, especially at younger ages. For example, a preschooler may be able to choose which toy to play with, but she may not be able to extend her evening play time beyond that allowed by her parents. A school-age child may be able to negotiate some extra play or computer time, for example, by proving that he has completed all his homework. An adolescent may be expected to organize her own schedule, within reason; so, the degree of choice is greater than for a younger child. Parents can make many choices for their children so long as they still live at home, but the ability to control or influence them gradually declines as they mature.

The second prerequisite for using problem solving is that no clear-cut rule exists that dictates what to do in the situation. Thus, it is not applicable to situations where there is a law or rule governing behavior. For example, you cannot choose to get on the bus and not pay your fare, as there are negative consequences for this behavior. You could, however, choose to take a nonstop express bus or a bus that makes all stops, depending on where you are going and how quickly you would like to get there. The number of situations without clear rules is increasing, however, as society changes more rapidly and becomes more complex than in previous generations. For example, new forms of communication on the Internet are developing almost weekly, with few rules to govern their use or abuse. Children are often among the first to access these new social opportunities and are well advised to stop and think about how to proceed. Thus, problem-solving skills are becoming increasingly important not just in dealing with therapeutic situations but also in mastering the day-to-day challenges of our current life.

Educators have been aware of the benefits of these skills for years and have used them to help students follow complex directions, solve mathematical problems, facilitate memory, improve reading comprehension, and develop other academic skills (Kendall & Bartel, 1990). They recognize problem solving as a means of active learning where the student must do something deliberate in order to learn rather than passively assimilating information that is provided. Active learning has consistently been found to be more effective than passive learning (reviewed in Schmidt, Cohen-Schotanus, & Arends, 2009). Thus, problem solving is an example of the old idea that "experience is the best teacher." Whether we are developing a manual skill like riding a bicycle or typing 60 words per minute, or correcting our behavior by remembering past mistakes, we use experience to learn. Furthermore, unlike facts we memorize for an examination and then forget almost immediately, things learned by experience tend to be retained. They stay with us, and we often consider them personal characteristics rather than things we once learned.

At the border between the realms of education and psychotherapy lie resiliency-focused programs, many of which are offered in school settings (reviewed in Noam & Hermann, 2002). The goal of these programs is to provide children without overt mental health problems (sometimes they have no problems; sometimes they have risk factors for certain problems) with skills to help them master life challenges. It is hoped that, as a result, the children will become less vulnerable to emotional and behavioral problems. Problem solving is a key component of most of these programs. This makes sense, as problem solving promotes independent thinking and builds confidence. Even if the teacher or therapist who engages in problem solving with the child does 95% of the work, the remaining 5% the child does becomes a new, encouraging experience for that child. Such encouraging experiences that demonstrate the ability to master challenges help children, and all human beings, develop confidence in their abilities.

WHAT IS THE EVIDENCE FOR THE BENEFITS OF PROBLEM SOLVING?

Problem-solving ability has been linked to a number of favorable mental health outcomes in children and youth. For example, skillful problem solving has been linked to better social functioning in youth at risk of psychosis (O'Brien et al., 2009), lower risk of depression in adolescent girls experiencing interpersonal stress (Davila, Hammen, Burge, Paley, & Daley, 1995), and improved adherence to diet in children with hyperlipidemia (Hanna, Ewart, & Kwiterovich, 1990). It may also protect at-risk adolescents from some forms of substance abuse, as problem solving has been found to mediate the relationship between adolescent hopelessness and lifetime alcohol and marijuana use (Jaffee & D'Zurilla, 2009). Conversely, poor problem-solving skills in adolescents have been linked to aggression (Greene, Ablon, Hassuk, Regan, & Martin, 2006; Kazdin, Esveldt-Dawson, French, & Unis, 1987a, 1987b; Lochman, Wayland, & White, 1993); self-injury and suicide attempts (Nock & Mendes,

2008; Wilson et al., 1995); depression, hopelessness, and suicidal ideation (Adams & Adams, 1996; Arie, Apter, Orbach, Yefet, & Zalzman, 2008; Carris, Sheeber, & Howe, 1998); and stealing behavior (Greening, 1997).

Family interactions related to problem solving may also affect mental health in youth. For example, families of teens with significant drug abuse showed negative problem solving interactions between parents and adolescents regardless of whether or not a drug-related topic was the focus of discussion (Hops, Tildesley, Lichtenstein, Ary, & Sherman, 1990). Adolescent–parent problem-solving style has been found to be related to adolescent–parent attachment style (Cobb, 1996), suggesting that addressing the attachment style may help in improving adolescent–parent problem solving.

Parent training may also play a role in improving problem solving in youth. Certain parenting behaviors have been found to predict cognitive problem-solving ability in children as young as 30 months old (Fagot & Gauvain, 1997) and social problem solving in adolescents (Reuter & Conger, 1998). In addition, maternal problem-solving responses to aggressive behavior in adolescents were found to be inversely related to the duration of the aggressive behavior (Sheeber, Allen, Davis, & Sorensen, 2000). Thus, when mothers responded to their aggressive teens by using a problem-solving approach, teen aggression subsided.

Given the many potential benefits of problem solving, clinicians and researchers have been eager to train children and adolescents in this set of skills. Surprisingly, the literature evaluating programs that promote problem-solving skills appears limited. However, this is likely attributable to the fact that problem solving is often considered a technique or therapeutic approach rather than a psychotherapy per se. Problem solving is a component of many therapies, and it is not always possible to tease out whether it is problem solving or another therapy component that accounts for the therapeutic change. In young children with disruptive behavior, for example, problem-solving training is almost always combined with parent training (Kazdin et al., 1987b), and it is not clear how much therapeutic change can be attributed to the child training versus the parent training. Nevertheless, a few studies reported in a large medical database (MEDLINE) evaluated programs based primarily on problem-solving techniques. These are summarized in Table 1.1. While the list may not be exhaustive, it does highlight the main populations for which problem-solving programs have been evaluated.

As the table shows, problem-solving training has been found most consistently to reduce externalizing behaviors such as aggression, dis-

TABLE 1.1. Therapeutic Benefits of Problem-Solving Interventions in Children and Youth

Population	Outcome	Reference
Child psychiatric outpatients	Reduced disruptive behavior	Michelson et al. (1983)
Institutionalized delinquent adolescents	Improved problem-solving skills, some generalization outside sessions	Hains & Hains (1987)
Children with antisocial behavior	Reduced antisocial behavior	Kazdin et al. (1987a, 1987b)
Depressed children ages 9–12	Reduced depressive symptoms	Stark, Reynolds, & Kaslow (1987)
Developmentally disabled youth	Increased appropriate social behaviors in work settings	Park & Gaylord-Ross (1989)
Adolescents with attention-deficit/hyperactivity disorder and oppositional defiant disorder	Reduced parent–adolescent conflict	Barkley et al. (2001)
Adolescents with elevated depressive symptoms	Reduced depressive symptoms	Spence, Sheffield, & Donovan (2003)
Aggressive child and adolescent inpatients	Reduced aggression; reduced need for seclusion and restraint	Greene et al. (2006)
Adolescents with traumatic brain injury and their families	Reduced internalizing behaviors, depressive symptoms, parental depression, parent–adolescent conflict	Wade, Walz, Carey, & Williams (2008)

ruptive behavior, and antisocial behavior. A few studies also suggest a beneficial effect on depressive symptoms, parent–adolescent conflict, and development of socially appropriate behaviors.

Even in this limited literature, however, there are some inconsistent findings. For example, Barkley, Edwards, Laneri, Fletcher, and Metevia (2001) studied teens with attention-deficit/hyperactivity disorder (ADHD) and found that parent–teen conflict declined with intervention, but only a minority of families (23%) showed reliable change. In younger children with ADHD, a large multisite study (Jensen et al., 2001) found that an intensive behavioral program that included problem-solving training was not significantly more effective than routine community care, unless the children were also given a carefully monitored stimulant medication. Perhaps the fact that children with ADHD have a neuropsychiatric condition can help explain these discrepant findings. Problem solving alone may not be sufficient to address behavioral problems in children with such conditions. This does not necessarily mean that problem solving is useless in children with neuropsychiatric conditions, but rather that it may need to be combined with other medical or psychological interventions in order for these children to benefit from it.

Similarly, there have been discrepant reports about the benefits of problem-solving therapy for depressive symptoms (reviewed in Bell & D'Zurilla, 2009). A recent meta-analysis concluded that problem-solving therapy was more effective when the treatment program included training in "positive problem orientation" (Bell & D'Zurilla, 2009) in addition to the standard problem-solving steps outlined below. In other words, negative cognitive biases about how soluble or insoluble a problem is may need to be addressed in depressed people before they can use problem solving effectively.

In summary, most evidence suggests that problem-solving ability in children and youth is associated with positive mental health outcomes, may protect oneself from certain negative mental health outcomes, and that training in problem-solving skills can reduce many mental health problems. However, in clinical populations problem-solving training may be more helpful if offered as part of a larger treatment plan tailored to the child's specific psychiatric disorder and individual needs.

AN OVERVIEW OF PROBLEM-SOLVING STEPS

Most of this book is organized in ways that relate to the key problem-solving steps shown in Figure 1.1. Note that the specific labels for these steps vary a bit among various problem-solving programs, but the concepts are the same across programs. After the next chapter detailing where and when one can use problem solving, subsequent chapters focus on each step. The chapters include discussion and examples of applications of each step to different age groups (within a 7- to 18-year range) and diagnostic groups (e.g., anxiety vs. ADHD). Common practice challenges related to each step are also described. Parents are often included in the problem-solving process, especially those who have younger children, but there is also a separate chapter on getting parents to continue at home what the therapist is doing in the clinic (a common therapeu-

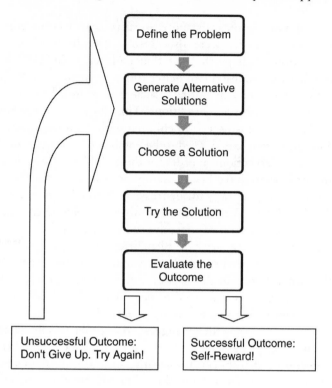

FIGURE 1.1. Problem-solving steps.

tic challenge). The remaining chapters describe how to combine problem solving with other interventions, teach problem solving in groups, and troubleshoot common difficulties encountered in this therapeutic approach.

To get an overview of what problem solving involves, let's look briefly at all five steps outlined in Figure 1.1 and see how they fit together by relating them to Mark's dilemma. Recall that Mark, the adolescent cited at the beginning of this chapter, was having trouble deciding about college. The first step Mark must take is to define the problem. At first glance, this appears obvious: he must decide where to go to college. If we think more carefully, though, we realize that his specific current problem is deciding to what college or colleges he will submit an application. The question of where he ultimately goes to college is not entirely within Mark's control. His father, his teachers, the college admissions committee, and perhaps other people can all influence that outcome. The problem of deciding which applications to submit, on the other hand, is one where Mark has at least some choice or influence. The only clear-cut rule he must follow is to meet the applications deadline, and this rule does not limit the type or number of applications he can submit. Thus, "Deciding which college applications to submit" appears to meet the criteria for a useful problem definition. Incidentally, problem solving is usually more effective when the initial problem definition is specific rather than general. In this case, the definition has the additional advantage of keeping Mark focused on the present task, which is manageable, rather than getting overwhelmed by the thought that he must design a plan for his whole education, perhaps his whole life.

Next, in Step 2, Mark must generate alternative solutions to his defined problem. He has already begun to do so in the example: he could submit an application to his father's alma mater, to the out-of-state college he is interested in, or to the local college with the good reputation. One possibility he may not have considered is to apply to all of them. Another possibility is to not submit any applications and decide to work or travel for a year after high school. Mark may need support in generating some of these alternatives because his anxiety about the decision may make it difficult to think about certain alternatives. "Brainstorming" (generating as many alternatives as possible without censoring oneself) tends to be easier in a calm frame of mind.

The third step is choosing a solution from among the alternatives generated in Step 2. To make the choice, Mark must examine the likely positive and negative consequences of each alternative. Sometimes it is also helpful to look at the short-term and long-term consequences for each alternative, as these may differ. If Mark chooses to write down his list of consequences, it might look something like this:

FATHER'S COLLEGE

- *Positives:* "Father will be happy, I don't have to deal with the stress of moving out of town, I will save money by living at home."
- *Negatives:* "I will be living at home and therefore have more rules to follow, I will be living at home and therefore be less connected to life on campus, I may miss out on a great program out of state, I may have to deal with people who knew my father in college, I don't know if they'll accept me."

OUT-OF-STATE COLLEGE

- *Positives:* "I may get a chance to pursue a great program, I will have more freedom from the rules at home, I may meet new and

interesting people, I will be more connected to life on campus, I won't have to deal with people who knew my father in college."
- *Negatives:* "My father will be upset, it might be scary to move so far away from home, the new people I meet might distract me from my studies, the 'great program' may not be all I hoped it would be, I will probably spend more money, I don't know if they'll accept me."

LOCAL COLLEGE

- *Positives:* "I don't have to deal with the stress of moving out of town, I will save money by living at home, there might be an interesting program there (don't know), I won't have to deal with people who knew my father in college."
- *Negatives:* "My father will be upset, I will be living at home and therefore have more rules to follow, I will be living at home and therefore be less connected to life on campus, I may miss out on a great program out of state, I don't know if they'll accept me."

This alternative highlights a common obstacle to problem solving, namely, lack of information. Mark may need to investigate the programs offered by this college before deciding whether or not to submit an application there.

APPLY EVERYWHERE

- *Positives:* "I don't have to deal with my father's reaction right now, I'm sure someone will accept me, I'll have more time to think about the final decision."
- *Negatives:* "I have to fill out lots of application forms, I have to deal with the uncertainty of not knowing where I'm going next year, I may again face the problem of deciding on a college in a few months if more than one college accepts me."

APPLY NOWHERE

- *Positives:* "I may become more confident by gaining some life experience, I don't have to worry about application forms, I'll have lots of time to decide on a college."
- *Negatives:* "It might be hard to start studying again after not doing it for a whole year, my father would never allow it."

This is quite an exercise! It also tells us something about Mark: any teen who can generate this number of possibilities is thoughtful and definitely not impulsive. Mark has a very good grasp of consequential thinking, but he's also quite anxious and may have trouble "seeing the forest for the trees" when examining his pros and cons for each alternative. Therefore, we are not going to have Mark do a meticulous tally of the number of pros and cons. Instead, we should ask him to look for recurrent themes or points of particular importance to him. For example, he repeatedly indicates that he doesn't want to deal with people who knew his father in college (a somewhat peculiar concern, but obviously important to him). The strong wording "my father would never allow it" also indicates that "apply nowhere" may not be a realistic option in this case. We should also observe how Mark reacts to each idea. For example, if he breathes a noticeable sigh of relief when writing down "someone will accept me," then that is a salient point for him that might help him decide. Finally, we must avoid the temptation to unduly influence Mark toward the choice we think best for him. The therapist's job is to help him decide, not to make the decision for him.

Assuming we have helped Mark choose a solution, he must now try it out. This means he must commit to a definite time and place to implement his solution, and also to evaluate the outcome. Scheduling a time for trying the new solution, or at least setting a time limit, is often helpful in ensuring that people try it. Old habits die hard, and most of us resist trying something new unless we commit ourselves to it. In evaluating the outcome, use as specific a measure as possible. "I will feel better after submitting the application(s)," for example, is a bit vague. "I will sleep an hour extra (or eat a healthier dinner, or complete my homework more efficiently, etc.) because I will be less stressed" is more specific.

If Mark's solution is helpful and he indeed feels less stressed, he should congratulate himself for solving his dilemma so thoughtfully and effectively! If his solution leaves him with continued stress, or perhaps worsening stress, it is important to not see this as a failure. Observe to Mark that it's common for people to "not get it right the first time," and encourage him to try again. For example, if Mark chooses to apply to the college out of state but then spends the whole night worrying about his father's reaction, this alternative may be difficult for him to live with even if it is consistent with his needs. Perhaps there is another solution that needs to be considered. Help Mark go back to Step 2 (generate alternative solutions) and then repeat the remainder of the steps until a satisfactory outcome is achieved. For example, perhaps applying to his father's alma mater in addition to the out-of-state college will reduce

Mark's stress. Alternatively, perhaps Mark needs to opt for a discussion with his father sooner rather than later to reduce the stress and worry about his father's reaction. Whatever his choice, if he tries it and finds himself feeling better, congratulate him and encourage self-congratulation too!

Mark's case is helpful in illustrating the steps of problem solving, but it is not necessarily typical. As mentioned, many young people are more impulsive than Mark or may need more guidance than he does to engage in the problem-solving process. Age, intelligence, diagnosis, family circumstances, and other factors can all affect problem-solving ability. On the other hand, the variety of challenges posed by these factors makes problem solving interesting. If every case were like Mark's, you might be tempted to stop reading at the end of this chapter. It is because of the myriad presentations and dilemmas we encounter in using this therapeutic technique with our young clients that it merits a book. Therefore, I invite you to read further!

Chapter 2

When and with Whom
Can You Use Problem Solving?

The preceding chapter emphasized the wide range of situations where problem solving can be a helpful therapeutic technique. You may be wondering if there are situations where it is *not* helpful. Indeed, although it is among the most versatile of therapeutic techniques, there are situations where problem solving is inadvisable. In this chapter, I examine some red flags that may indicate that problem-solving is likely to be difficult or ineffective, at least as an initial strategy. Here is an example of a case where problem solving was ineffective.

Shortly after graduating from my training program in psychiatry, I was referred an 8-year-old boy, Jackson, for psychotherapy. Jackson had been in several foster care placements since the age of 3, when he was removed from his parents' home owing to evidence of repeated physical abuse. About 6 months before I met Jackson, his father had obtained a court order permitting supervised visits with his son. Since the visits began, Jackson's behavior at school and in his foster home had deteriorated dramatically. He often had angry outbursts, was inattentive in class, and had been accused of bullying several kindergarten children.

Jackson said little to me initially but became more animated when discussing the games of his favorite basketball team. After a couple of sessions of discussing basketball, I decided to see if Jackson was interested in doing some problem solving regarding the situations where he typically got into trouble (e.g., losing his temper at school and bullying others). He said that he would like to get into trouble less often and that he thought the bullying would be easier for him to stop than the temper outbursts. I started asking him details about situations where he had bullied other children to see if he could respond differently in those situations. He reported that he bullied "crybabies" and "wimps" who didn't fight back. He went on to say that he just "roughed them up" and that "they don't know what real pain is." He became increasingly agitated as he spoke. Unfortunately, I then wondered aloud if memories of his own experiences of pain might be connected to his anger toward "wimps." At this point, he became enraged, pushed over a table with papers on it, and threw a small chair in my direction. I ducked, suggested he take a break in the waiting room, and restored my office to its former state.

The next week, we talked basketball. The following week, I made another attempt at problem solving, again with destructive results, and this time Jackson ran out of the office and into traffic. Fortunately, he was not harmed. I then arranged a meeting with Jackson's foster parents and a Children's Aid worker, where I shared my impression that a stable home and more limited contact with his father would do more for Jackson's mental health than individual psychotherapy. I offered to continue to be available as a consultant to the foster parents and the worker but to defer therapy until Jackson's place of residence and parental visits had stabilized and he began showing some capacity to trust others.

Although I sometimes wonder if Jackson would have done better with a more experienced therapist, he was certainly not an ideal candidate for using a problem-solving approach. There were several red flags that suggested this case would be challenging. These will be discussed further below as I consider factors in the client, the family, the therapist, and the therapeutic relationship that may interfere with using problem solving successfully. Before doing so, however, it is worth checking whether there are findings in the psychotherapy literature relevant to the question of treatment suitability when using a problem-solving approach.

FACTORS FOUND TO AFFECT PROBLEM-SOLVING THERAPIES

Problem solving can be the primary focus of psychotherapy or simply one of several treatment components. If it is the primary focus, standardized manuals for the problem or population of interest are often help-ful. For example, Philip Kendall's (1992) *Stop and Think Workbook, Second Edition,* has been designed for preadolescent impulsive children. Such manuals usually spell out the characteristics (e.g., diagnostic pro-file, age, gender, academic ability) of children or youth that benefit the most from their use. If problem-solving is only one of several treatment components, the criteria for using it are less stringent, but there are still some factors that predict an easier or more difficult course. Some of these relate to general readiness for psychotherapy, while others relate to specific characteristics of the child, family, therapist, or therapeutic relationship.

Studies of adults with various forms of substance abuse have formed the basis of a common and often useful model of readiness for psycho-therapy, the readiness to change model, initially proposed by Prochaska and DiClemente (1984). This model can be used by therapists of diverse theoretical backgrounds. It posits that clients are more likely to ben-efit from psychotherapies, especially action-oriented therapies like those focused on problem solving, if they are further along a series of stages the authors describe. The initial stages (precontemplation and contem-plation) involve recognizing one has a problem and beginning to consider addressing it. Later stages (preparation and action) involve more active planning and implementation of new behaviors. Clients in these later stages are considered better therapeutic candidates than those in the ear-lier stages. The final stage (maintenance) involves consolidating the new behavior and making it an ongoing habit. If the client is in one of the ini-tial stages, the therapist must work on enhancing his or her motivation to change before proceeding to problem solving or other action-oriented interventions. Clients can also move back and forth among the stages or cycle through the stages several times in the course of developing new behaviors (Prochaska, DiClemente, & Norcross, 1992). They may also be more ready to change one behavior than another.

In adults, there are various standardized measures of readiness to change (see Ogrodniczuk, Joyce, & Piper, 2009). These are not com-monly used in child psychotherapy, but one can still look for signs of readiness to change in initial interviews with children and parents. In youth, one must assess the parents' readiness to change their behavior toward the child as well as the child's readiness to change. Thus, an anxious parent might say about his or her child that "I want her to be more independent" (contemplation stage) but label independent behav-iors attempted by the child as dangerous or foolish. For example, I have seen teens that were told to be more independent but were not allowed to use public transit, go to the library, or go to a friend's house unless accompanied by an adult.

Some questions that may facilitate a discussion of readiness to change might include the following:

- "What could you/your child do differently in this situation?"
- "What would be a different approach to this problem?"
- "What do you think another person in your/your child's situation might do differently?"
- "Would you/your child be willing to try that different behavior/ approach? Why or why not?"
- "What would stop you/your child from trying a different behavior/approach?"
- "What have you/your child tried in addressing this situation/ problem so far?"
- "Why do you think what you/your child have tried so far hasn't worked?"
- "What else could you/your child try? Do you think it could work? Why or why not?"
- "What would be a small sign that the situation was starting to improve?" (Note: this question is useful because people need to be able to notice signs of progress in order to persevere with new behavior.)

Being alert to the stages of change in children and families is particularly important when the treatment referral is initiated by people outside of the immediate family. Jackson's therapy referral, for example, was initiated by the Children's Aid Society with little regard for Jackson's wishes or those of his foster family. Well-meaning school personnel also often initiate referrals for assessment and treatment of children with mental health problems. Sometimes these are helpful, but at other times families feel stigmatized by having their child identified as having a mental health problem and will either not follow up or will follow up but undermine the treatment in some way. Cases from these sources are not necessarily impossible to treat, but they usually require some initial sessions focused on treatment motivation with the child and family (see Brody, 2009, for a description of motivational interviewing with adolescents).

A few studies have examined specific factors that may affect the success of problem-solving interventions with children and families. Higher cognitive ability has been linked to more successful problem solving in adolescents (Frank, Green, & McNeil, 1993; Siegel, Platt, & Peizer, 1976), although results are not entirely consistent. In the sample of Siegel et al. (1976), for example, emotional problem solving related to intelligence but social problem solving did not. They hypothesized that emotional problem solving requires more abstract reasoning than social problem solving, accounting for its stronger link to intelligence. Therapist factors may also affect the success of problem-solving interventions. For example, a qualitative study of general practitioners using problem-solving therapy for depression found that, while they had broadly positive attitudes toward the therapy, some feared losing personal control of their consultations, resulting in potentially adverse patient outcomes (Pierce & Gunn, 2007). Time constraints in a busy practice were also cited as a potential barrier to using problem-solving therapy. Finally, high levels of family conflict have been cited as potentially interfering with problem-solving-based interventions (Adams & Adams, 1996).

Beyond the factors that have been studied empirically, however, we can examine readiness to engage in problem solving based on what we know about the technique. This examination is summarized in Table 2.1 and will now be described with respect to the client, the family, the therapist, and the therapeutic relationship.

THE CLIENT

Once you are confident that the child and family are ready to work toward changing their approach to a particular problem or situation, it is important to clarify where problem solving fits in the overall treatment plan. An effective treatment plan depends on an accurate diagnosis and a formulation of the factors that are contributing to the child's mental health difficulties. In Jackson's case, for example, a diagnostic assessment might have uncovered posttraumatic stress symptoms related to his past abuse and/or ADHD. A formulation would have almost certainly hypothesized difficulties with trust and close attachments, stemming from early exposure to an abusive parent and repeated disruption of attachments to foster parents as he was moved from one placement to another. Recent reexposure to the formerly abusive parent (his father) and reminders of the abuse (by an unwary therapist) could heighten these difficulties, accounting for his increasingly disruptive behavior and his violent reaction in therapy.

Using this more thorough understanding of possible reasons for Jackson's misbehavior, one could then plan for treatment. The plan

TABLE 2.1. Signs of Readiness to Begin Problem Solving

The client

- Readiness for change/alternative behaviors
- Clear diagnosis, formulation, treatment plan
- Some influence on the situation(s) addressed
- Minimum cognitive and communication ability to participate in problem solving
- Has skills to do alternative behaviors
- Able to come for consistent appointments

The family

- Readiness for change/alternative behaviors
- Able to come for consistent appointments
- Able to bring child consistently
- Limited family discord
- Empathy for child's dilemma
- Willing to give child some choices about situations addressed

The therapist

- Willing to give child and family some choices about situations addressed
- Able to book consistent appointments
- Confidence in ability to use problem solving successfully
- Empathy for child's/family's dilemma
- Able to adapt problem solving to child's developmental level

The therapeutic relationship

- Time taken to establish rapport
- Collaborative (everyone has a say; everyone has a part to play)
- Transparent
- Agreement to talk about specific problem(s) repeatedly

Contraindications

- Severe conduct disorder or unsafe situation requiring urgent attention
- Problem completely outside child's control
- Recent crisis in the family, limiting the child's control over his or her life
- Child has severe cognitive distortions affecting problem solving
- Diagnosis resulting in symptoms that interfere with the ability to participate in psychotherapy (e.g., selective mutism; can still problem-solve with the family in this case)
- Severe cognitive limitations and/or lack of communication ability (can still problem-solve with the family in this case)

would need to consider which of Jackson's difficulties ought to be addressed first: posttraumatic symptoms, inattention, aggressive behavior, or mistrust and attachment problems. Because the ability to trust another human being is such a basic requirement for therapy, I elected to prioritize this issue. Given his foster parents' firm but caring approach and their ongoing day-to-day contact with Jackson, I thought they were most likely to gain his trust. Once able to fully trust them, Jackson might be able to trust a therapist in the future. At that time, problem solving regarding the behavioral issues might be possible, though additional therapy would likely be needed to address the posttraumatic symptoms.

Like Jackson, many children and adolescents who struggle with a problem-solving approach do so because they have psychological problems that interfere with their ability to use it. Therefore, if there is another evidence-based treatment that is indicated for the diagnosis of the child you are seeing, pursue this alternative approach first. Problem solving may still be indicated later in the treatment plan or in combination with the other treatment. It can be particularly helpful for addressing the real-life challenges that sometimes result from having had a psychiatric illness. For example, a boy recovering from depression may struggle to explain to his peers why he missed a term of school; or a girl who is recovering from panic disorder may not know how to deal with her friends' reaction if she has an attack in front of them; or a child with medically treated ADHD may wonder how to reassure others that he will no longer impulsively break their toys.

Let's assume for the moment that you are considering using problem solving with a child who has a clear diagnosis, formulation, and treatment plan, and (unlike Jackson) is able to tolerate psychotherapy sessions without too much distress. What other characteristics would the child need for problem solving to succeed? Considering each problem-solving step in turn, the child would need:

1. To be struggling with a problem or situation where he or she has at least some influence on the outcome.
2. To have enough cognitive and communication ability to think about and talk about alternative behaviors. (Note: the therapist can assist with both generating alternatives and selecting the best one.)
3. To have the skills needed to perform the alternative behaviors.
4. To come back for follow-up appointments to review progress and adjust the problem-solving plan if needed.

The Child's Influence on the Outcome

The first of these requirements depends on the age and developmental level of the child. Thus, an 8-year-old (or a developmentally delayed 12-year-old) might be able to make her own lunch by putting together a bologna sandwich and pouring a glass of milk, but expecting her to use the stove to cook a hot lunch might be unrealistic or even unsafe. Thus, the problem to be solved should be phrased as "preparing my own lunch" rather than "preparing a hot lunch."

Sometimes other people must be involved in solving the problem. For example, if an 11-year-old is obese, he might say, "I need to do a sport to become more fit," and proceed to think about different sports he likes more or less. Unless his chosen sports are running or biking, though, he needs to consider when and where the sports are available and who can transport him to the practice sessions. Since he is too young to drive, his parents will likely need to be involved in the problem-solving discussion.

The Child's Cognitive Ability

The cognitive and communication ability needed for problem solving is not extensive, so long as the therapist can adapt his or her work to the child's abilities. Even children who are too young to do formal problem solving can be prompted to develop the logical and creative thinking skills needed. For example, one might use such prompts as "How many things can you think of that are green?" or "What else could you do in this situation?" for creative thinking skills; or "What would happen if you did X?" for logical/consequential thinking skills. A preschooler may need the therapist to guide and contribute ideas during each step, while a 7- to 12-year-old might just need the therapist to provide prompts for each step (if he or she lacked the ability to combine the steps independently), and a teenager may be able to problem-solve fairly independently if the therapist provides meaningful praise and encouragement.

Let's look at a few examples. The phrases in brackets provide reminders as to which problem-solving step is being addressed.

PRESCHOOLER EXAMPLES

STACY: I keep getting into trouble for forgetting my mittens at school.

KM: Would you like to figure out how to keep track of them? [defining the problem]

STACY: Sure! Then my mom would stop yelling at me.

KM: So ... where could you keep the mittens so you don't forget them?

STACY: I dunno.

KM: How about your coat pockets or inside your hat? [suggesting alternatives]

STACY: Last week, I lost my hat *and* my mittens!

KM: So, do you think the coat pockets might work better? [evaluating alternatives and facilitating making a choice]

STACY: Yeah. I guess so.

KM: Could you give that a try? [implementing a solution]

STACY: Sure, if I remember.

KM: Is it OK if I ask your mom to remind you?

STACY: OK. And can you ask my teacher too? [suggesting another means of implementing a solution!]

KM: Good idea! I'll ask them both to remind you, but you should try and remember too. Then, next week, you can tell me how it's going. [setting a follow-up time]

In this case, I facilitate every step of the process for Stacy, but she participates willingly and even contributes an idea at the end. I positively reinforce this, in order to send the message that her contribution is valued and to encourage her to contribute even more to future problem-solving discussions.

JACK: Nobody plays with me in the playground.

KM: Would you like to figure out how to get them to play? [defining the problem]

JACK: OK.

KM: What do you do now when you want someone to play with you? [eliciting alternatives]

JACK: (*shrugging shoulders*) I dunno. I guess I walk up to them.

KM: And then?

JACK: I stand around, but they never ask me to play. They always ask another kid.

KM: Is there anything else you could do? [eliciting more alternatives]

JACK: I dunno.

KM: What do other kids do when they want to play with someone?

JACK: I guess they say "Can I play?"

KM: Could you do that? [evaluating alternatives]

JACK: They might get mad 'cause they don't know me.

KM: So ... you might need to tell them your name first, and find out their name. That way, they would know who you are.

JACK: (*blushing*) I don't think I'd do that.

KM: You look nervous about that. Let's practice what to say a few times here. Then, when you're comfortable, you can try it in the playground. Does that sound OK? [suggesting learning a skill so he can implement a solution]

JACK: (*becoming teary*) I don't want to. I wish I could just have friends!

KM: I wish I could do magic and get you some. Shazam (*waving an imaginary wand*)! Oh, dear, I don't think that worked. But learning to play with kids may be a good way to start making friends. Is there even one kid who plays with you already? [redirecting to the problem at hand]

JACK: Yeah, there's Rob from next door, but he's not at the playground most days.

KM: Do you think your parents could talk to his parents and get you guys together more? Would you be OK if I asked them to do that? [suggesting another solution and offering to implement it]

JACK: OK. My mom sometimes talks to his mom anyway.

KM: Thanks, Jack. I'll talk to your parents today and let you know what they say. [reinforcing his cooperation and agreeing to follow up]

In this case, Jack is anxious enough that he is not even willing to *rehearse* approaching other children; so, I guide him toward a solution that relies on grown-up help. It's not ideal since it does not allow Jack to solve the problem himself, but it is a realistic first step. If Jack had been less anxious, I would have role-played some approach behaviors with him and then determined whether or not he needed adult support when trying them out.

SCHOOL-AGE EXAMPLES

JASON: Whenever I try to start my project I get distracted and do something else. [defining the problem]

KM: Let's figure out how to settle down and get to work on it. OK?

JASON: (*sounding skeptical*) All right ...

KM: What do you do when you try to start the project? [prompting a clearer description of the problem]

JASON: I open my books, boot up the computer, pull out my notepad, and sharpen my pencils.

KM: Sounds good. Then what happens?

JASON: I see a game on the computer I really like, or sometimes my friends are on MSN, and then after a while I get hungry and have a snack, and then I see that my favorite show is on and ... I never get back to the project.

KM: So the computer, which is supposed to help with your project, sometimes ends up distracting you.

JASON: Yeah, I guess so.

KM: What things could you do to avoid that problem? [eliciting alternatives]

JASON: I could do the parts of the project that I don't need the computer for first, or maybe I could use a computer that doesn't have any games or MSN on it. [generating two alternatives]

KM: Could you try one or both of those ideas? What do you predict would happen? [prompting consequential thinking and making a choice]

JASON: I think that could work. My teacher always says I should do an outline first anyways before I look up stuff online. I could ask my mom about her computer too, and I think it would be OK because she doesn't use her computer in the evening much. My dad's computer has more games on it than mine, though! (*Laughs.*) [evaluating alternatives and thinking about implementing his solutions]

KM: Sounds like a plan! Give it a try, and you can tell me next week how it went. [reinforcing his choice and willingness to implement, indicating follow-up time]

As you can tell, Jason is taking more responsibility for his problem than a younger child would and is contributing more ideas to the problem-solving process. The therapist's job is to prompt each step and to positively reinforce his participation.

> CARRIE: (*animated*) Kathy used to be my friend, but then I saw her kind of whispering with Karen. I'm not sure if they were whispering about me or Sally, 'cause Sally used to be Karen's best friend until she got invited to Rachel's party and went, because nobody likes Rachel, you know ... So now I'm not sure if Kathy is still my friend. Maybe I'll ask Jennifer what she thinks. She used to be friends with Kathy before I was, and she can't stand Karen. What do you think?
>
> KM: I've got to admit, I'm confused. That's quite a soap opera! How do you keep track of all those people and what they all think about each other? [acknowledging my limitations and helping her define the problem]
>
> CARRIE: It's not easy! (*Laughs.*) But that's just the way it is at my school.
>
> KM: Does anyone ever give you a straight answer? [further problem definition, with some empathy]
>
> CARRIE: Not really. Do you think I should just talk to Kathy? [suggesting an alternative]
>
> KM: That might be the simplest thing to do. Are you OK with that? [I check if she is ready to implement the alternative, or we need to look at another solution.]
>
> CARRIE: Yeah, she's pretty easygoing. I'll just catch her after class tomorrow. [making a choice and a plan for implementation]
>
> KM: OK. Let me know how it turns out. [informal suggestion of follow-up]

Carrie's dilemma, by the way, does not constitute any particular psychopathology. Clandestine social interactions among fifth-grade females are common, and often confusing!

TEENAGE EXAMPLE

> JENNIFER: My parents won't let me stay out with my friends. They say we're irresponsible, just because they caught us sharing a beer once.

KM: So, I guess we need to figure out how to get your parents to trust you enough to let you go out with your friends again. [defining the problem]

JENNIFER: Can't you just tell them to let me go? They always listen to doctors. [proposing an alternative]

KM: I'm not going to be there every time you disagree with them though, Jennifer, so I think in the long run it makes more sense to figure out how you can get them to listen to your point of view. [evaluating the alternative and proposing another one]

JENNIFER: (*sarcastically*) My parents listening? That's a joke!

KM: Your friends are important to you, though, so maybe we should brainstorm some ideas of what you could say to your parents. Even if they only listen on this one issue, I think it would be worth it. Do you?

JENNIFER: OK. But I'm not going to lie!

KM: I don't think you have to. I think your parents worry about you being safe when you're out with friends. What are some things you could say to reassure them that you'll be safe? [reframing the problem so it is more within Jennifer's control: reassuring parents is more feasible than making parents listen or making parents change their minds]

JENNIFER: I could take my cell phone and tell them I'll call home if there's a problem or if I need a ride. I could tell them I'll be back by curfew. I could tell them where we're going and who's driving. I could take some money so I can get a cab if I need to. I could even get some of my friends to pick me up so they can meet them and see that they're not a bunch of stoners or anything. It seems like a lot of trouble to go to for a night of fun, though ... but I guess if it gets my parents to loosen up I should try it. Can I ask them here, at the end of the session? I wasn't kidding when I said they listen to doctors. They'll be much more reasonable in front of you. [lots of alternatives, willingness and plan for trying them, request for limited support]

KM: OK, I can bring them in, and you can tell them your ideas. I can't promise they'll change their minds, but I'll try to make sure they listen until you're finished. Let's see how that goes. [clarifying the proposed solution, with a plan to evaluate the outcome]

Jennifer presents a common teen dilemma: ironically, she wants to depend on the therapist to help her become independent of her parents. Instead, I suggest an alternative way of negotiating autonomy from her parents and then prompt her to find her own ways of talking to them. This suggestion results in a more age-appropriate approach and avoids my being drawn into the parent–teen conflict. Jennifer generates most of the specific ideas to solve her problem, once she is convinced that the problem has a solution that is within her own control. Similarly, Mark (the teen in Chapter 1) also generated most of the ideas needed to solve his problem. He still benefited from the therapist's guidance, however, in sorting through the merits of various options he was considering.

To summarize, therapists offer most of the problem-relevant ideas when working with preschoolers, help with organizing the process in school-age children, and offer guidance as needed in adolescents.

There are further examples throughout the book on how to do problem solving with different types of children. However, children who are nonverbal or selectively mute (i.e., do not speak to the therapist because of their social anxiety) may have difficulty with problem solving regardless of the therapist's abilities.

The Child's Having Sufficient Skills to Solve the Problem

The skills that may be needed for problem solving depend on the specific problem, but common ones include social skills, academic skills, athletic skills, and rules for popular games. Some aspects of these skills may be taught by using problem solving (see Kendall, 1992), but a few basics usually need to be memorized. For example, problem solving could be used to help a child develop an approach to solving mathematical word problems, but addition and subtraction facts have to be learned by rote. Similarly, figuring out how to make a new friend may be amenable to problem solving, but knowing not to stand too close to someone is a basic social rule that must be learned.

The Child's/Family's Ability to Plan for Follow-Up

Finally, problem solving requires at least one follow-up visit after the initial session to make sure that the child has tried the new behavior that was agreed upon and to evaluate the result. Even if the result is positive, the child benefits from positive reinforcement from the therapist, and this increases the likelihood of the new behavior's continuing. If the result is not positive, it is even more important to review what happened, with the goal of either choosing a new alternative or trying again. Either way, the therapist can encourage the child not to give up. Of course, if problem solving is the primary focus of therapy, multiple sessions will be needed. With adolescents, it is important for the teen to be advised of the need for follow-up session(s) and to be convinced of their value. Younger children are reliant on parents bringing them to therapy, so the need for follow-up should be emphasized with families in this case (see below).

THE FAMILY

Because children are less self-sufficient than adults, family characteristics affect the likelihood of success with a problem-solving approach. Some of these characteristics are needed regardless of one's therapeutic approach with the child. The family must be ready to change their behavior toward the child or at least accept that the child may behave differently. The same questions listed above for assessing the child's readiness to change can also be asked of the parents. The ability to come consistently for appointments and to bring the child consistently are important as well, given the need to follow up and evaluate the success of any new solution that is implemented. Of course, families struggling with their basic needs (e.g., difficulty feeding their children or difficulty finding or maintaining affordable housing) sometimes cannot make children's mental health appointments a top priority. Mental health services providers that can go into the home are sometimes needed in these circumstances. Families where parents struggle with their own mental health problems can also have difficulty attending appointments consistently.

Families that are highly conflicted or have difficulty empathizing with their child's dilemma can undermine even the best psychotherapy. It is sometimes hard to judge whether family therapy is needed first, before attending to the child's needs, or whether psychotherapy with the child should be given the priority. If family members cannot remain in the same room together for a full session without being verbally abusive to one another, family therapy should probably come first. On the other hand, sometimes increased problem-solving ability in the child can reduce family discord. For example, I once saw a recently separated and highly conflicted family where the older boy's ability to juggle school work with looking after his younger brother (a plan arrived at by problem solving) enabled his mother to work and make a successful separation from her abusive husband. Thus, family conflict should not be considered an insurmountable obstacle to a problem-solving approach.

Parental empathy is particularly important for younger children, for whom solutions are highly dependent on their parents' participation. Parents who say "My child just needs to suck it up," or something similar, are highly unlikely to support new solutions to the child's problems. These parents may need other types of counseling first (either family therapy or, alternatively, psychotherapy that addresses parents' interpersonal or attachment styles). For adolescents, while a lack of parental empathy may hurt the teen emotionally, nonetheless he or she may still be able to solve his or her problems independently.

One issue that is unique to problem-solving approaches is the need for the family to be willing to give the child some choices about situations addressed in the work. Children typically have more limited choices than adults do, but as they progress toward maturity they need to make some choices in order to learn adaptive adult behaviors. For example, a child may not be able to choose how to get to school at age 7, but by 12 he or she may be able to take the bus independently. Families that are unwilling to allow this behavior may undermine the child's confidence and ability to use public transit into adulthood. I once worked with a family of a teen girl with a well-controlled seizure disorder who were very anxious about this issue. Eventually, they were able to allow their daughter short trips on the bus, so long as they had arranged for an adult to meet her at her destination. Similarly, the family of a child with a severe peanut allergy would not let him go on school field trips, but once they were reassured by extensive education of the school personnel, including practice with an EpiPen (used to administer epinephrine), the child was allowed to participate.

Another variation on the "anxious family" theme is the family that insists on doing everything for the child. For example, parents may say, "She doesn't need an allowance, we buy her everything she wants or needs," or "We don't believe in children doing housework." In both cases, the child may be very comfortable but later on may encounter special difficulties in moving away from home, as he or she has never learned to manage money or has never learned to do laundry, cook, or do other common household chores.

Besides anxiety, cultural factors may also limit the autonomy parents are willing to grant their children. For example, the family of a child from a strict religious background would not let her go to movies with her friend. She was allowed out of the house only if chaperoned by a parent or older brother. Working within these cultural parameters can be challenging but possible if one reminds the parents of the long-term goal: to have their child function as a successful member of the local community.

Occasionally, parents may pay lip service to a problem-solving approach but balk at its implementation. These parents are not really interested in seeing their child change, but rather are hoping for a more placid, compliant child. They may make statements like "That's nice, dear—aren't you clever?" and then ignore the child's efforts to implement a new solution. In these families, it is often worth asking the parents, "How would your life be different if he (or she) no longer had this problem?" Find out the negative as well as the positive consequences of solving the problem. These negative consequences may make the parents resistant to helping the child implement new solutions. Work with the parents to see the long-term benefits to the child (and perhaps also to themselves) of solving the problem.

THE THERAPIST

The therapist as well as the client needs to be ready to use a problem-solving approach. The most common difficulty therapists face is the inability to prescribe a "right" answer for the client. Because problem solving is truly collaborative, the therapist must accept that the client may end up choosing a solution the therapist considers inadvisable. This relative lack of control over the client's progress is often disconcerting. For example, the therapist may worry about being held liable for the client's "bad" choices. So long as those choices are not attached to a legal requirement, however (e.g., the requirement to report impaired drivers, or persons likely to harm themselves or others), they must be respected. Consistent follow-up ensures that any problematic choices will be evaluated and adjusted with the client. Consistent follow-up may be difficult in a busy practice, however. Illustrating this dilemma, general practitioners have identified discomfort with the therapist's relative loss of control as being implicit in problem-solving therapy (Pierce & Gunn, 2007).

Therapists with extensive training in other modalities unrelated to problem solving may also experience discomfort. For example, therapists with analytic training may denigrate problem solving as an overly concrete or superficial approach to psychological issues, while therapists with cognitive therapy training may feel limited by the problem-solving approach, as it focuses on actions rather than thoughts and feelings.

THE THERAPEUTIC RELATIONSHIP

Establishing rapport and a trusting therapeutic relationship is an essential prerequisite for a problem-solving approach. Children often require a few sessions to get to know the therapist, to share common interests, and to trust that the therapist has their best interests at heart. Being clear about the limits of confidentiality (i.e., that the therapist can only keep confidential those things that are not likely to be harmful to the child or to another person in the child's life) is important in working with clients of all ages. Being clear about the extent of therapist–parent contact and what will or will not be shared with parents is equally important.

Finally, the problem to be solved must be important to the child, not just to those surrounding the child. Children's therapy is often initiated by concerned parents or teachers with little regard for the wishes of the child. The child must come to see that there is a personal benefit to working with the therapist beyond that of merely appeasing upset parents or teachers. If the child is eager to solve one problem and the parents want to address another, I usually advise the parents to be patient. The parents' issue will be addressed eventually, but making the child's concern a priority improves the chances of developing a good therapeutic relationship with the child and thereby avoiding premature termination of the therapy.

CONTRAINDICATIONS

In some situations problem solving is not appropriate or helpful. For example, in the case of Jackson at the beginning of this chapter, problem-solving attempts made matters worse. Some other situations where problem solving may not be helpful or where other interventions should be attempted first include:

- Severe conduct disorder (problem solving may help the child escape the consequences of his or her actions but will not change the disorder).
- A child who is too cognitively limited to participate in problem solving (as noted earlier, this limitation applies only to children below the preschool level of cognitive functioning).
- A child who has severe cognitive distortions that preclude accurate perception of the problem. For example, an intelligent but

depressed child may say, "I can't talk to my teachers about catching up on my school work. I'm stupid. I just can't do it!"

- A clear cause for the problem that is outside of the child's control. For example, a child who is being severely bullied and cannot defend him- or herself really has only one option, namely, to tell an adult who can put a stop to the abuse.
- A selectively mute child who won't communicate in sessions, even nonverbally. These children often need a combination of medical and nonmedical treatment to increase their ability to communicate outside of the immediate family (Manassis, 2009). Problem solving becomes relevant once they are able to engage in some verbal interactions with the therapist, but prior to that point the focus needs to be on increased social speech, regardless of the other problems they are facing. The family may be able to engage in problem solving together with school officials, however, to facilitate progress (Manassis, 2009).
- A recent crisis that is outside of the child's control. For example, recent family separation issues may make the child upset, and associated family financial stress may reduce the activities the child can do, but the focus in this case needs to be on the grown-ups reestablishing some stability in their lives. The child can do little to improve this situation.

Despite these obstacles to problem solving with children, this type of intervention is still possible in many situations. One must think about the overall treatment plan, however, and determine where and when interventions focused on the child, including problem solving, are likely to be most helpful.

Chapter 3

Step 1: Defining the Problem

After deciding that a problem-solving approach is likely to be helpful in a clinical situation, it is tempting to immediately talk to the child and family about a clear definition of the problem to be solved. Taking a moment to discuss the *nature of problem solving* with the child and family, however, can often help avoid difficulties later. Having a clear idea of *one's role as a therapist* before starting is also worthwhile, as it can make the problem-solving process more predictable and less daunting. These two issues are now discussed before detailing how to define a "good" problem to be solved.

CHILD AND FAMILY EXPECTATIONS
OF PROBLEM SOLVING

Problem solving involves experimenting with new ideas and behaviors in a thoughtful manner. That is, the child and therapist think beforehand about which solutions to the problem are more likely or less likely to be helpful, and they evaluate afterward how helpful or unhelpful the selected solution actually was. Families sometimes believe that the approach is either not sufficiently experimental or thoughtlessly or randomly experimental. Both of these opinions are troubling.

In the first case, the family may think that the therapist will provide the child the illusion of choice while actually orchestrating the process behind the scenes. "The doctor will fix the problem (or fix the child)" is an unspoken assumption in this case. There is often a further assumption that therapeutic progress will be smooth and quick, as it is entirely dependent upon the "expert" therapist. It is important to explain that the child will be allowed to try solutions the therapist may not consider optimal. However, any solution that is clearly dangerous (e.g., running across train tracks in order to catch a train) will be discouraged, and the parents will be informed if their children or teens disclose a desire to harm themselves or others. Otherwise, though, the child will be allowed to learn from experience. Some families are anxious about the possibility of the child's making mistakes. This should be discussed openly. Sometimes it is reassuring to them if it is pointed out that people of all ages learn more effectively from experience than from books or lectures, and as well that the therapist is open to hearing about their concerns at any time during the therapy. At other times families cannot be sufficiently reassured, and then problem solving may need to occur at a later time or be focused on the parents rather than the child.

In the second case, worry over excessive experimentation, the family may assume that "anything goes." In other words, the child will try out different ideas that may or may not be helpful, with no thought beforehand or afterward, until he or she happens to find a solution that works. The problem with this assumption is that it minimizes the roles of both the therapist and the parents in guiding the child through the process step by step. For this family, it is important to spell out the ways in which they can support the therapy and the child's progress. Bringing the child to appointments regularly, modeling effective problem solving for the child, being aware of the therapist's role (see below), and positively reinforcing the child's new behaviors can all serve to support the therapy and therapeutic progress.

Finally, some families bring an underlying pessimism to the process. They may agree to therapy with reluctance, saying, for example, "I guess it's worth a try. Nothing else has worked," or "Sure, go ahead, doc. Maybe you'll have better luck with her than we've had." In this case, it is important to be clear with the family that you are not denigrating their previous efforts to help the child or claiming to be especially clever in your work with children. Rather, you are providing an opportunity to try out new behaviors, some of which may have even been tried before, in a new context. That new context involves carefully thinking about what is likely to work, whether the new behavior needs to be combined with other interventions or supports in order to work, doing it very consistently, and then evaluating progress systematically week by week. The level of planning, monitoring, and consistency involved in the process is more rigorous than what most families do when trying to solve problems in their day-to-day lives. Therefore, although success cannot be guaranteed, the chances of success are higher than in previous attempts to solve the problem.

A further source of pessimism is sometimes found in the assumption that therapies that do not address the "root causes" of problems cannot be effective. Families with this assumption may believe that their child's problems relate to deep-seated conflicts or traumas that have not yet been discovered, and that such discovery is essential for their child's behavior to improve. In this case, it is important to show the family that a careful mental health assessment of the child has been done and to provide a description of the conclusions of that assessment, including likely factors contributing to the problem. Then, gently provide the family with a summary of empirical evidence for therapies that do not address "root causes" (e.g., therapies based on problem solving, behavioral therapy, or cognitive-behavioral therapy), emphasizing any studies relevant to their child's particular problem. Some families are convinced by this evidence to try problem solving, while others seek further mental health assessments for their child. Either way, you have challenged an important assumption that could otherwise undermine therapy.

THE ROLE OF THE THERAPIST

How the therapist goes about teaching problem solving to children and adolescents is summarized in Figure 3.1. Some aspects of the therapist's role are described in greater detail in Phillip Kendall's (1992) *Stop and Think Workbook, Second Editon*. Refer to the steps in Figure 3.1 as I describe the role of the therapist.

Modeling

To begin, the therapist models a problem-solving approach to a problem that is obvious to both the child and the therapist. Kendall (1992) emphasizes that it is important to do "coping modeling." In other words, the therapist models making mistakes and coping with them, in addition to modeling successful outcomes for the child. For example, suppose that the child and therapist are both looking at the following word puzzle:

"Find the name of a mammal in the following letters: *B T I B R A*."

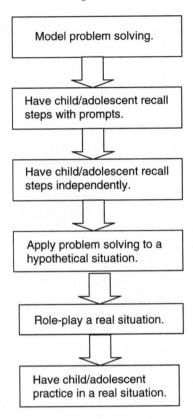

FIGURE 3.1. Therapist's steps in teaching problem solving.

The therapist models:

"Let's see, now. I think I need to unscramble some or all of the letters to find the name of the mammal [defining the problem]. I need to take my time and look at all the possible answers [looking at alternatives]. Then, I focus in on my answer: I think it's a bear [choosing a solution]! Let's try that [trying out the new solution]. Oops! Bear is spelled *BEAR*, not *BAIR*. I got it wrong [evaluating the result]. Oh, well, everyone makes mistakes sometimes. I'll just try again [coping modeling]. I'll look carefully at the letters for other answers. Another answer might be ... rabbit. Let's try that. OK, *RABBIT* works. I got it right. It's good that I persevered [evaluating the result and self-reinforcement]!"

Notice how slowly and carefully the therapist proceeds. This slowness is deliberate, to reduce the chances of the child's impulsively choosing an undesirable or ineffectual solution. Also notice that the therapist has started with a word puzzle rather than a problem related to emotions (the latter being one of the more common reasons that children are brought to therapists). This is also deliberate. Problems that do not relate to emotions are often perceived by children as less threatening than those that do, and beginning with a word puzzle also allows for engagement with children who have a limited vocabulary for emotions (see below regarding developmentally appropriate language).

This example also illustrates that problems can have more than one correct solution. A clever child (or adult) will notice that *BAT* is also a mammal whose name can be found in the scrambled letters. Thus, the example can also be used to allow the child to "teach" the therapist or to encourage the child to find multiple solutions. Both are likely to boost the child's confidence and problem-solving ability.

Parents can model problem solving for everyday problems around the house to further familiarize the child with the process. For example, I have long known that I do not have a particular talent for doing home repairs and therefore usually avoided dealing with them in the past. Nevertheless, after being widowed several years ago, I found myself one day confronted with a toilet that would not flush. My son alerted me to the problem and asked, "What are we going to do?" As he listened, I talked myself through the problem something like this:

> "This [expletive] thing won't flush! What do I do with it [defining the problem]? I could call a plumber, but they take days to come and cost a fortune [looking at alternatives]. I could try to fix it myself, but if I get it wrong I could end up flooding the house. Maybe I can open up the back of the tank, see what looks broken, and describe it to the old guy at the hardware store. He could probably tell me what to do or at least tell me if I need a plumber or not. That's what I'll do [choosing a solution]!"

I went to the store, described what I saw in the back of the tank, and was told I needed to replace a part that cost only $3.50. I bought the part, did as I had been told, held my breath, and flushed [trying the new solution]. It worked perfectly, and I exclaimed, "Great! Who would think I could actually fix something around the house! I'll do that again if I need to do another unexpected home repair [evaluating result and self-reinforcement]." I was rather pleased with myself, and my son was reassured that his mother could manage a minor home repair without too much distress by doing some logical step-by-step problem solving. Modeling thus increased the chances of his resorting to problem solving when faced with his own dilemmas in the future.

Teaching the Steps

After being exposed to some modeling of problem solving, including coping modeling, the child or adolescent should be encouraged to learn the required steps. Have the child or adolescent put the steps into his or her own words. For example, "alternatives" may become "different choices" or "possible answers"; "evaluating the result" may become "ask myself how I did" or "ask myself if it worked." The child should be able to recall the steps, initially with some prompting or "clues" provided by the therapist and later independently.

Next, the steps are applied to several hypothetical situations. Usually the therapist presents these, but some children or adolescents are able to suggest some situations that "could happen someday" or that "happened to a friend." Note that the latter situations are sometimes not so hypothetical, as children and teens will sometimes use the expression "it happened to my friend" as a way of getting advice about real problems in their lives. In this case, I usually don't challenge the real versus hypothetical distinction but keep in mind that the problem may need to be revisited as a "real situation" in a future session.

As the child or adolescent becomes more proficient at problem solving with hypothetical situations, he or she can be encouraged to address real ones. It may help to role-play the new solution(s) during a therapy session first, to make it seem less threatening in real life. This is particularly true of social situations where new skills are needed. For example, an adolescent who wants to address the problem of loneliness at school by introducing himself to someone in the cafeteria may need to role-play common conversation starters; similarly, a child who wants to ask her teacher for extra help may need to learn how often it is OK to ask for help during class and when a separate meeting with the teacher is needed.

Implementing New Solutions

Finally, new solutions must be tried outside the office in day-to-day life. Some children need the support of either a parent or the therapist to implement a new solution, while others do not. Adult support makes it more likely that the new solution will be tried consistently, but it also reduces the child's ability to learn from mistakes and to gain confidence from trying a new behavior independently. Some judgment is needed regarding the degree of adult support. In younger children, I usually inform parents of what the child is planning to do, the degree of support the child does or doesn't want from them, and whether I think this is appropriate. If there is little risk associated with the situation (e.g., a child wants to try a new way of approaching a problem with a teacher), I usually let the child decide. If there is some risk (e.g., the child wants to stand up to a bully who has hurt him or her in the past), I may advise parental support. Many adolescents prefer to address day-to-day problems independently; so, I usually respect their confidentiality and do not inform parents of their choices without first asking for permission. However, if the situation is clearly dangerous (e.g., there is a risk of self-harm or harm to others), I inform the parents regardless of the adolescent's wishes.

Another part of having the child or adolescent try new solutions in real life is helping him or her identify all the situations where these solutions are relevant. Some children may not recognize similarities between situations, making it difficult for them to generalize a new solution across similar situations. This is a particularly common problem for children with certain learning disabilities. For example, a child may reassure herself that she will see her parents again soon when waiting for them to come home. However, she may not realize that the same self-reassurance could be applied when she has to leave her parents to go to school. The therapist may need to point out that both situations involve a separation between parent and child and therefore the same strategies can be applied to both. Another child may have learned to cope with getting less story time when the evening routine is running late but still explode when he gets French toast instead of pancakes for breakfast. Both situations involve things being "slightly different from usual" and thus might respond to similar strategies, but the child may need help in identifying this similarity.

Defining the Problem

Developmentally Appropriate Language

In order to define a problem in a way that is clear to both the therapist and the child or adolescent, both need to speak the same language. I don't mean that they must necessarily speak English, or Spanish, or some other formal language, but they must have a common way of discussing emotions and behavioral or emotional problems that both can understand. As therapists, we easily slip into professional jargon, often without knowing it. Adults may find this annoying but still usually understand what we mean. Children often do not. In Table 3.1, I have outlined some therapists' expressions and the corresponding colloquial expressions that children and adolescents may be more familiar with. This list is not exhaustive, and colloquial expressions change frequently, but it is a starting point for thinking about some terms that may allow clearer communication with your youngest clients. Once the therapist and the child or adolescent are using common terminology, the specific problem to be solved can be defined in these terms. Some examples are listed in the table.

Baseline Severity

If possible, try to quantify the severity of the problem so that, after trying a new solution, you can objectively measure any change. Recording the

TABLE 3.1. Getting the Language Right

Therapist's jargon	Child/adolescent equivalent
Managing anxiety	Being less nervous, not getting stressed out, not being scared, coping with stress
Reducing aggressive outbursts	Controlling my temper, keeping my cool, calming down, cooling off, taking a breather, counting to 10, chilling
Positive reframing/ positive self-talk	Looking on the bright side, seeing the silver lining, seeing the glass half full, affirmations, thinking positively
Self-reassurance/ coping self-talk	Thinking realistically, getting a grip, getting real, taking some perspective, believing in myself
Behavioral activation	Getting more active, getting some exercise, doing more things every day
Exposure	Facing my fears, being brave
Generalized anxiety disorder	Being high-strung, being uptight, being tense all the time, being a worrywart
Social phobia	Being too shy, getting tongue-tied or stage fright, getting embarrassed easily
Clinical depression	Feeling low all the time, being really moody, being "emo," being down in the dumps, having a nervous breakdown

baseline severity of a problem enables one to notice small signs of progress week by week. This is encouraging for both the client and therapist. How does one quantify severity? Try to identify what would constitute small signs of improvement in the situation you are addressing. Perhaps the child gets through the situation with less disruptive or less emotional behavior. Perhaps the child acts more quickly, or perhaps more slowly but more accurately, successfully, or with greater confidence. Many children can also rate the difficulty of a situation or distress experienced in a situation on a scale from 1 (easy) to 10 (very difficult or distressing). Again, try to use the child's terms to quantify severity as to well as define the problem.

WHAT CONSTITUTES A "GOOD" PROBLEM TO WORK ON?

The facetious answer to this question is that, by definition, a problem is never "good." What the question is really asking, though, is what constitutes a good focus for a problem-solving approach in therapy. Goffin and Tull (1985, p. 28) described four characteristics for such a focus:

- The problem must be interesting and meaningful to the client.
- The problem must be solvable in more than one way.
- The problem is one that requires or allows for a new decision.
- The outcomes of the new decision can be evaluated.

Difficulties finding a "good" problem usually relate to at least one of these characteristics. I have already discussed the need for families and children to understand and agree to a somewhat experimental approach, which implies that multiple solutions exist and will be considered. The need to evaluate the severity of the problem and how it changes in relation to the new solution (or decision) has also been described. This leaves us with the task of defining what constitutes an "interesting and meaningful" problem. But perhaps it is easier to define what sorts of problems are often *not* perceived to be interesting and meaningful. In my experience, these can include:

- A problem that is vague or nonspecific.
- A multitude of problems that cannot be reduced to a single focus.

- A situation that is not perceived to be a problem by the client.
- A situation that is not perceived to be amenable to change by the client.

Let's examine each of these in turn.

Nonspecific Problems

In order to solve problems effectively, it helps to focus on those that relate to specific situations. For example, it is easier to solve the problem "How do I effectively ask my teacher for help in math class?" than "How do I improve my grade in math?" The first problem immediately brings to mind various ways of getting the teacher's attention, politely asking for clarification of particular ideas or questions, and perhaps arranging a time to meet with the teacher after class if the child or adolescent is still confused. The second problem requires more thought because it is broad and really consists of several component problems relating to study habits, ways of asking for help, determining if tutoring is needed, and so on.

Parents and children can both present overly vague problems to the therapist. Sometimes, this relates to wishful thinking. Recall the example of Jack in the preceding chapter who wanted to "just have friends." This lofty goal is unlikely to be amenable to a situation-specific approach like problem solving. Parents often engage in wishful thinking with respect to change in their children. "Just give him self-esteem" or "Help him behave better" or "I want my child to be more motivated at school" or "I want my child to stop feeling shy" are examples of such wishful thinking. Here, the parent is hoping for a change in temperament, personality, or diagnosis but has no idea how to bring that change about.

Guiding children and parents to think about specific situations that relate to the problem they present is often helpful. Thus, the therapist could ask Jack if he had ever had a friend before, and if so, how that friendship first started. Then, Jack could think about putting himself in similar situations to make more friends. If there were no previous friendships, the therapist might ask "Where could you meet someone who might become a friend?" and explore what he might do in that situation. In the case of the parents' complaints about the child, the therapist could ask when and where the child characteristics they describe are adversely affecting the child's life or the parents' lives. After one or more specific situations are described, the problem can be reframed with respect to those situations.

Sometimes children and parents feel discouraged when told that the problem must be solved one situation at a time. In response, the therapist can reassure them that their problem-solving skills will improve with each situation they work on. Thus, progress may be slow at first, but once they have mastered several related situations they will become more confident and the process will speed up.

Another reason for children and parents presenting overly vague problems relates more to memory than wishful thinking. Some people have very clear situation-specific memories known as "episodic memories" (Tulving, 2002). Other people remember many general ideas about the past but few specific situations. For example, one child may say, "Geography is hard for me," while another says, "On my last geography test, I got confused and I ran out of time. Then, I panicked and couldn't finish—so, I got a really low mark." To begin problem solving, the second description is much more helpful. It immediately leads to developing alternative strategies for taking tests and managing test-taking anxiety. In the first description, it is not clear if the child has difficulty understanding geography concepts, reading the geography textbook, completing geography assignments, or taking geography tests.

Fortunately, most children and parents who remember general ideas can also remember specific episodes if prompted to do so. "Can you think of a particular time when you realized that geography was hard for you?" or "When was the last time that you struggled with geography?" are examples of questions that can prompt memories of specific episodes. If the child is still struggling to remember specific situations related to the presenting problem, sometimes one or both parents can remember them. If all family members have difficulty recalling specific episodes, having them keep a daily diary of problematic situations can help. This may seem like a chore initially, but within a week or two it usually clarifies which situations must be tackled.

A Multitude of Problems

Sometimes children or parents have already spelled out half a dozen problems by the time you tell them to slow down and focus on one thing at a time. Anxiety, learning or attentional difficulties, and really having a large number of challenging problems can all result in this dilemma.

Children or adults who tend to worry a great deal (when extreme, this is called "generalized anxiety disorder") will sometimes worry that things cannot improve if the therapist does not have an absolutely complete picture of their difficulties or those of their child. They often bring lists of problems to sessions and are dismayed when told that only one or two items on their list will be addressed initially. They may question the therapist's ability to help them if not allowed to finish describing all of their difficulties in detail. They may also look for unrealistic guarantees regarding the success of therapy or request to see only the most "expert" therapist in the clinic. Rather than responding to these demands defensively, it is usually helpful to describe the therapeutic relationship as a collaborative one and to emphasize that you are not able to help anyone who is not willing and able to participate in the process.

Then, ask them to prioritize their concerns. For example, you could ask, "What is the one daily situation where your life or your child's life is most difficult?" or "When in the past week have you or your child been most upset by these issues?" Adding a time frame of "daily" or "in the past week" encourages people to focus on specific situations that are currently relevant to their lives. If people continue to describe multiple problems, I sometimes take them through a typical day, from the time they wake up in the morning to the time they fall asleep, to get a clearer idea of when and where they are facing significant problems and what those problems are. Prioritizing concerns in this way is also helpful for clients who are unable to focus on a single problem because of distractibility or inattention.

Children with certain learning disabilities can sometimes present multiple problems and not realize that they all relate to a similar theme. This difficulty is particularly common in children who have nonverbal learning disabilities or are on the autistic spectrum. To these children, getting angry when asked to get off the computer is perceived as a completely different situation from getting angry when asked to switch from one subject to another at school. The fact that both situations involve sudden transitions from one activity to another is not obvious to the child. Therapists can be helpful to these children by listening to their various concerns for a period of time, sometimes a few sessions, and then, depending upon the child's cognitive abilities, either identifying or helping them identify one or more common themes. Problem solving can then be applied to one situation consistent with that theme. Later, the successful solution can be applied to the other situations consistent with that theme.

Finally, some families face multiple realistic challenges in their lives. When they describe multiple problems, many of them may not even relate to the child's mental health. Housing, employment, transportation, child care, hunger, and neighborhood violence may be among their many problems. In this case, you may choose to collaborate with colleagues in social service agencies who can help address these realistic challenges before attempting problem solving that is focused on an emotional or behavioral issue. If the family is motivated to address the emotional or behavioral issue, however, it is possible to attempt both concurrently. In this case, it is important to ensure that the child and parent(s) can attend sessions consistently despite the other problems, and that they realize that as a therapist you can only help with the emotional or behavioral issue(s). For example, providing bus tokens may do more to ensure therapeutic success than any particular psychological technique for these families.

"No Problem," According to the Client

When a child reports having "no problem," I rarely take this response at face value. Usually, the child is trying to avoid talking about problems. Some children are concerned about appearing vulnerable, and so, they deny problems in order to appear strong. In this case, explore with the child what he or she thinks happens to people who appear weak or vulnerable, and ask whether the child has been victimized when appearing this way. Normalizing problems can also help. Give examples of problems many children of similar age face, and, if appropriate, disclose one or two problems you yourself have faced. When the child realizes that everyone has problems from time to time, the possibility that he or she has one does not seem so threatening.

Some children claim to have "no problem" because they are either oppositional or unhappy about being brought to therapy. I recently worked with an 11-year-old girl, Sally, who presented in this way.

> KM: Can you think of an example of a situation that was tough for you this week?
>
> SALLY: (*silent shoulder shrug*)
>
> KM: Was there even one situation like that?
>
> SALLY: Nope. I dunno.
>
> KM: Your dad mentioned you seemed tense on the way to the appointment today. Is something bothering you?
>
> SALLY: (*silent shoulder shrug*)
>
> KM: What would you rather be doing right now?
>
> SALLY: Not missing my math class!
>
> KM: I thought you didn't like math.

SALLY: Yeah, but when I miss it I don't understand the homework, and then I get in trouble with the teacher the next day for not doing it.

KM: No wonder you're tense! I think I'd be worried too. Is there anything you can do so you don't get into trouble tomorrow?

SALLY: I dunno.

KM: Would it help to talk to the teacher at the start of the class?

SALLY: I guess so.

KM: What would you say?

SALLY: That I couldn't do my homework because I missed the class for a doctor's appointment, so I didn't understand.

KM: Do you think she'd listen to you?

SALLY: Probably. But I'd still be pretty far behind.

KM: Could you do part of the homework?

SALLY: Maybe. My teacher usually gives part marks if we show we tried to do the work.

KM: Sounds like a plan! Let me know next time how it went.

SALLY: Do you think we could do a later appointment next time?

KM: Maybe, but we need to check your dad's schedule too.

We checked, and it was feasible to see her an hour later; so, she did not miss math class repeatedly. Working with Sally became easier and less tedious after she was reassured that she would not repeatedly miss the same subject.

One further possibility to consider regarding the child who claims to have "no problem" is that he or she is hiding something. Children trying to protect secrets will often feel the therapist is prying if asked directly about problems. For example, a child who is being bullied and has been threatened with violence if he or she tells an adult may have many emotional or behavioral symptoms but report "no problem." The same may be true of children who are physically or sexually abused. Some children are forced to protect other secrets—for example, their family being in the country illegally or being involved in illicit activities. In certain cultures, there is also a great deal of stigma attached to emotional or behavioral problems, and at times some suspicion of mental health providers. In this case, there may be no family secrets, but children may still be encouraged to claim they are "fine" even when they are upset.

The Perception That Things Cannot Change

The perception that the problem is not amenable to change is particularly common when one or more people in the family are depressed or dealing with an overwhelming life stress. For example, I remember working with a mother and her 14-year-old daughter who were struggling to deal with the death of a son from a chronic illness several years earlier. The mother presented the problem as "My daughter isn't going to class, and I don't know what to do. My son would never have behaved this way. I guess it's just the way she is." The father worked long hours and did not attend the appointment.

Inquiring about the family's home life, I discovered that the mother had made a virtual shrine of her son's room, went to church daily to atone for the "sin" of not saving his life, and saw herself as being punished by God for not being a better mother to him. A few months after his death, this behavior might have been considered part of the grieving process. Three years after his death, it clearly represented more significant psychiatric illness (likely depression) on the mother's part.

The daughter had been referred for psychiatric assessment because of school truancy that was thought to be anxiety-related (as I work in an anxiety clinic). When interviewing her, it quickly became obvious that her truancy had nothing to do with anxiety. Rather, she was sitting in a donut shop near the school with her friends, eating and smoking and talking about her life. She felt completely ignored at home because of her mother's preoccupation with her dead brother; so, she found an emotional connection with others by spending time with like-minded peers who felt equally neglected. Her behavior was quite adaptive, given the problems she faced at home. Thus, it was unlikely to change until she could reconnect with at least one of her parents.

In this case, I did not elect to do problem solving with the daughter but rather referred the mother for assessment and treatment of her depression and tried to increase the father's involvement with his daughter, especially in helping with schoolwork. With some coaching from her dad, she returned to class and was eventually able to graduate.

WHEN PROBLEM DEFINITIONS DIFFER AMONG THE CHILD, PARENT(S), AND PROFESSIONALS

Ideally, the problem to be solved should be defined the same way by the child, the parent (or parents), and the therapist or other professionals involved. Thus, there are at least four potential sources of discrepancy:

discrepancy between the child and the parent(s), discrepancy between the child and the therapist, discrepancy between the therapist and the parent(s), and discrepancy among professionals. In two-parent families, the parents may also disagree with each other, and divorced or reconstituted families where three or four adults are involved in parenting the child present even more complex possibilities. For simplicity, let's examine the child–parent, child–therapist, therapist–parent, and interprofessional discrepancies only. It is important to resolve these discrepancies because helpful new solutions are unlikely to be generated and implemented consistently if the people most involved in the child's life cannot even agree on the nature of the problem.

Sometimes, discrepant views on problems can be resolved by prioritizing (see below). Thus, one person's main issue is addressed first, and the other person's second. When the relationship is fairly amicable, this often works well, as people are willing to wait their turn when reassured that their issue will be addressed eventually. More serious discrepancies usually result when people define problems in terms implying that others need to change rather than focusing on what is within their own control or sphere of influence. Examples of this type of discrepancy are illustrated under the four specific headings below.

Child–Parent Discrepancies

> MOTHER: Jeff [age 12] doesn't do any homework unless I constantly remind him. He even lies about not having homework. He needs to work on his study habits! Can you help him with that?

> KM: Let's hear about the homework situation from Jeff's point of view first. Jeff?

> JEFF: Mom never says anything when I finish my work or get a good grade, but if I have one little bit of stuff left to do she's all over me ... like "When are you going to do it? Why haven't you done it yet? Why can't you be more responsible like your sister?" She won't even let me watch the hockey game on days when I don't have homework! She doesn't believe me, or she says I need to review even though the test is a month away. She needs to stop nagging me and get a life!

> KM: (smiling) OK, so it sounds like we're aiming for more homework and less nagging, right? (Mother and Jeff agree.) Jeff, is there anything you could do to reduce the chances of your mother nagging you? [redefining the problem in terms of what he can control]

JEFF: I have no idea.

KM: Do you think your mom nags more or nags less when you tell her you don't have homework and she finds out later that you do?

JEFF: More, I guess. She gets real upset when that happens.

KM: And Mrs. H., since they haven't discovered a homework gene yet, what do you think you could do to help Jeff improve in this area? [redefining the problem in terms of what she can control] It sounds like the constant reminding hasn't worked very well.

MOTHER: I give up.

KM: It sounds like there's so much emotion around this issue, we're not even clear how much homework is or is not getting done. Why don't we take a week to get a clearer picture of what is happening. Jeff, could you show your mother the homework you finish every night this week if she promises not to say anything about it? Mrs. H., I know you might have to bite your tongue, but could you live with that? (*Both agree.*) Then, next time we can talk about what we think a reasonable amount of work would be and the kind of feedback that might motivate Jeff.

In this case, the parent and the child have very different views of the problem, but it is essentially the same problem: a negative parent–child interaction around homework that interferes with its completion. For that reason, I chose to tackle both stated problems at once rather than trying to prioritize them.

Child–Therapist Discrepancies

Children often hope that their therapist will intervene on their behalf with family members, teachers, peers, or other people in their lives. Some social conventions foster this idea (e.g., the need for a "doctor's note" when children miss school or other activities for a period of time). Nevertheless, the more children can find their own solutions to problems, the greater their sense of confidence and personal competence. Therefore, I usually aim for a problem definition that recognizes the child's ability to influence the situation. Here is a common example: the tormenting sibling.

ALLISON (age 9): Can you tell my parents to punish Bobby [age 7], not just me, when we fight? They always say I'm older so I should know better, but it's not fair! He takes my stuff, he goes into my room without asking, he hogs the remote so we only watch his shows, and he calls me names behind Mom's back. Then, if I do anything, it's "Stop that, Allison. Don't you treat your baby brother that way!"

KM: That must be very frustrating. It's too bad we don't have a video camera at your house so your mom could see all the stuff that happens with you and Bobby.

ALLISON: I know. I never have proof of what he does. She only sees me blow up, and then it's always my fault.

KM: That must feel awful. Too bad I don't have proof either, so ... I'm not sure it would help for me to tell her this stuff. Is there anything you could do differently the next time this happens?

ALLISON: I try to ignore him, but I can't! (*tearful*)

KM: (*sympathetically*) Maybe there are other things you could do. Do you remember the last time this happened? If we go through what happened step by step, maybe we can figure out some other things you could have done and try those next time. Does that sound OK?

Allison agreed, and soon she was able to identify the common ways her brother "pushed her buttons" and either leave the situation or approach her mother at that point, before there was a big "blowup." I did some education about sibling issues with her mother as well (e.g., that a 2-year age gap does not necessarily imply greater maturity in the older child). Then, we focused on helping Allison to find ways of controlling her temper around Bobby. We all feel better when we have some ability to control our negative emotions.

Therapist–Parent Discrepancies

Mr. and Mrs. J. were a quiet, reserved couple who had a somewhat rambunctious 10-year-old son, Kyle. I had done a thorough psychiatric assessment of Kyle (including interviewing his parents), and apart from the difference in temperament between Kyle and his parents there was no evidence of any significant psychiatric problems.

MR. J.: Our 10-year-old son, Kyle, has been getting into more trouble at school. He's very bright, but he's so immature! He passed a cartoon he drew of the teacher to one classmate, he shot rubber bands at another, and he even pulled up his shirt in front of a girl! My wife and I don't understand why he behaves that way. We talked to him, but he couldn't explain his feelings. He's not very forthcoming in describing his emotions. We know he must be troubled, but even the play therapist he saw recently couldn't seem to get to the root of the problem. Can we work on discovering what motivates Kyle's behavior?

KM: You've just said that Kyle doesn't talk much about his feelings, and that's unlikely to change, at least in the short term. Thus, I'm not sure you will have much luck discovering his motivations.

MR. J.: Well, perhaps you could get through to him. You've worked with children like Kyle before, haven't you?

KM: Yes, I have, but in my experience trying to pry into their feelings and motivations is not always helpful, especially when there is a plausible explanation for the behavior. If I were a very bright but immature boy like Kyle sitting in a classroom, I think I'd be bored, and goofy behavior is pretty common among bored 10-year-old boys. The question is: How can we reduce the behavior that is getting Kyle into trouble and find a healthier outlet for his natural intelligence? Do you have any thoughts?

MR. J.: But, but ... he exposed his chest in front of a girl! Surely that can't be normal!

KM: Is the girl still upset? Is the school pursuing it any further?

MR. J.: No, thank goodness. She's fine and the school seems to think it's an isolated incident.

KM: Then let's assume this was Kyle's way of relieving boredom and maybe drawing some attention to his plight. You can still have a consequence for behavior like that, and you might want to discuss that with your wife, but we should also see if Kyle can be given some more challenging things to do at school

MR. J.: What about his lack of communication about his feelings?

KM: Once his boredom and his behavior improve, you may both have more positive feelings to discuss. Positive feelings are often easier to start sharing than negative ones.

At this point, Mr. J. agreed to the behavioral approach to his son's difficulties I had outlined, reassured that opportunities to discover and discuss his son's feelings would arise eventually.

Discrepancies among Professionals

These discrepancies often occur if more than one professional is involved in a child's mental health care and the professionals do not regularly communicate, or if a mental health professional and school official have different perspectives on a problem. The latter situation might occur if temporary accommodations at school are needed as part of a mental health treatment plan but the school sees this as indulging the child or allowing parents to be overprotective.

> PRINCIPAL: Hello, doctor. Mrs. M. is still dropping off Suzy right at the school door every day and taking her home for lunch too. Suzy is 8 now, and children of that age are usually allowed to be more independent. Can you talk to this mother about backing off a bit?
>
> KM: I appreciate your efforts to help Suzy with independence, but a couple of months ago Suzy was so anxious she was not attending school at all. Having her mother accompany her has allowed her to return and should serve as a stepping stone toward coming to school on her own. I'd like to see her become more independent too, but it may not happen overnight.
>
> PRINCIPAL: When do you see it happening?
>
> KM: After a few more small steps. For example, if Suzy arrived with her mother a few minutes before school starts, could one of your staff meet her in the school yard so she is less concerned about her mother leaving her there? Could she be assigned a peer "buddy" who could do this? Those are just some of the possibilities. I think Suzy's mother is also interested in fostering her daughter's independence. Would it be possible for me to meet with you and Mrs. M. together?

The principal agreed to the meeting, and reframing the problem as "fostering Suzy's independence in small steps" (which everyone could work toward) rather than "getting Mrs. M. to back off a bit" (which neither the principal nor I could control) was helpful in getting everyone to work together toward a common goal.

PRIORITIZING PROBLEMS

Sometimes children face multiple problems that require therapeutic attention and that are amenable to a problem-solving approach. Consider the example of Chad.

Chad was a 12-year-old boy who lived in a single-parent household. His mother worked in housekeeping in a local hotel, and also at a local dry cleaning store to make ends meet. He had two younger sisters who teased him mercilessly until he lashed out at them. Then, Chad would be the one to get punished for losing his temper. He was on the school basketball team, but his coach indicated that he could not continue unless his grades improved. Chad tried to study, but he was easily distracted and often forgot his books at school. When he came home, he remembered he was supposed to finish an assignment, but by then the school was closed and he could not get his books. At bedtime, Chad was supposed to make his sisters go to sleep, but they pranced around on the beds until their mother came home. She was usually exhausted and angry with Chad for falling behind at school and for not keeping his sisters in line. Chad was getting discouraged, angry at the unfairness of his situation and depressed.

This example raises an obvious question: Where should the therapist start? As a rule, it is more effective to start with easier problems and work up to more difficult ones. Doing so builds confidence as the child experiences repeated success. In this case, coming up with alternatives to the bedtime routine (or lack thereof) and finding a way to help Chad remember his books might be helpful and relatively easy. Assessing Chad for depression and possible ADHD would take time to arrange and be more complicated for the family, given the need for his mother to work at two jobs. The sibling issues could also be addressed better, but these would be unlikely to resolve until Chad's mother had more time for all three of her children.

When there are two relatively easy problems and one is more important to the child while the other is more important to the parent(s), the clinician must use some judgment as to which one to start with. If the parents are impatient, they may not continue to bring the child to therapy if their main issue is not addressed quickly. If the parents are able to wait, however, it is ideal to start with the child's main issue. Children have a more limited perception of time than adults. A 40-year-old may be reassured when told that her issue will be addressed in a month or two. By contrast, a school-age child could interpret "a month or two" as an eternity. He may remember what happened last week and look forward to the coming weekend, but anything beyond next week would seem meaningless.

Sometimes two problems can be addressed concurrently, especially if the child and the parents can work in parallel. In the example above, Chad's mother could do some problem solving on the bedtime routine while Chad could focus on getting school supplies better organized. Difficulties can arise, however, if the parents become frustrated by a lack of progress with what they consider to be the main problem or if they are unable to positively reinforce progress with what the child considers to be the main problem. In this case, it is better to stop trying to address both problems and decide which to address first.

I decided, in Chad's case, to speak to the teacher about a day planner in which Chad could be reminded to list his homework assignments every day and to provide a bag into which Chad could put his books each day whenever he realized he would need one for his homework. As his homework completion improved and he was able to continue on the basketball team, Chad became more hopeful about his future and his family situation.

Having read in this chapter about all of the preparation needed to do problem solving, from correcting families' expectations of the process to accurately defining and agreeing upon the best problem to start with, you may be thinking "Let's get to the creative solutions already!" This is a natural reaction, and it will be addressed in the next chapter. Before doing so, let me provide one word of caution, though. Do you remember the "BAIR" example from the word puzzle at the beginning of the chapter? Leaping to solutions too quickly, whether one does so in therapy or in real life, is not helpful. One of the greatest merits of a problem-solving approach is its tendency to slow down the thought process, allowing a more considered response. This is particularly helpful when working with impulsive children, but people of all ages can benefit from proceeding "one step at a time."

Chapter 4

Step 2: Generating Alternative Solutions

When we see children and families struggling with problems, it is obvious that what they have been doing so far to improve the situation hasn't worked very well. There is a need to look at other ways of doing things, other options, or alternative solutions. If these effective alternative solutions were easy to find and to implement, they would probably already be in place. The fact that they are not in place suggests that either they are difficult to think of or difficult to implement. In this chapter, I examine how to go about generating effective alternatives. Implementation will be discussed in a subsequent chapter.

After discussing how to encourage children to generate alternatives and some age-related differences, I examine such common challenges as children who have difficulty generating alternatives, children who see only one solution, children who generate too many alternatives, parents who do not consider certain alternatives, clients who want you to provide the alternatives/solutions, dealing with dangerous or concerning alternatives, and accepting when there is no alternative. The common practice of giving one a "choice within limits" is also examined.

BRAINSTORMING

The process of thinking of alternative solutions to a problem has commonly been termed "brainstorming." It has been studied in various age groups and in relation to numerous problems, with interesting results. For example, people sometimes question whether thinking of more ideas necessarily results in better ideas. Nevertheless, when judged by originality, feasibility/utility, or effectiveness, the quality of ideas resulting from brainstorming appears to be related to the quantity of ideas produced (Dornburg, Stevens, Hendrickson, & Davidson, 2009; Muato & Adainez, 2005; Tsukamoto & Sakamoto, 2001). Furthermore, brainstorming appears to be equally or more effective when done with individuals than when done with groups. Dornburg and colleagues (2009), for example, recently found that individuals and groups produced a comparable quantity of ideas when brainstorming, but the quality of ideas was higher for individuals. Pleasure in task performance has been found to mediate the quality of the ideas produced (Tsukamoto & Sakamoto, 2001), reminding us of the importance of picking problems that are relevant to the child and encouraging brainstorming in the context of a good therapeutic alliance where it is experienced as engaging and fun.

MODELING HOW TO BRAINSTORM

The word *brainstorming* may conjure up images of a hurricane or blizzard, and the analogy of a storm is a good one. To generate alternatives, people need to allow their minds to engage in free—even turbulent—patterns of thought. Thinking in the familiar patterns they are used to is unlikely to generate many new ideas.

When encouraging children to generate alternatives, modeling our own capacity to do so is important. Children respect people who "walk the walk" rather than just "talking the talk." For example, if I need to cancel an appointment, I might problem-solve out loud by saying, "Changing that appointment will surely be inconvenient for your parents, Trudy, so I hope they're not too upset. I suppose I could explain the reason for the change, though, and they may understand. I could also offer to squeeze in an extra appointment the following week if the new time doesn't work. Maybe I could also get their e-mail address so that I can let them know sooner if this ever comes up again." Then, I would make precisely these same suggestions to Trudy's mother or father and proceed from there. Trudy gets the message that even grown-ups have problems, perhaps making her less embarrassed about discussing her own. She also learns that there are many possible solutions to problems that can make them more manageable, but that most people need some time to think of these. Hopefully, she will see the value of taking time to think of alternatives in dealing with her own problems. If not, I (the therapist) can remind her of this example later when addressing one of her problems.

IS THERE A NEED TO GATHER
MORE INFORMATION FIRST?

When you examine alternatives and then select one, it is crucial to have all the information relevant to the problem. Remember the plumbing example in the preceding chapter? I needed to gather information from the clerk at the hardware store before I could decide whether to call the plumber or attempt to fix the toilet myself. In this case, selecting the best alternative depended on having accurate information. Similarly, it may be helpful to provide children and families with information relevant to their emotional or behavioral issues before they attempt new solutions to problems. For example, anxious children and their families often benefit from learning that solutions that involve avoiding anxious situations often make the anxiety worse in the long run. Only by facing their fears can children overcome their anxieties. Parents of children with behavior problems may benefit from learning that setting limits without becoming emotional is usually more effective than yelling at the child.

In other situations, information gathering is needed before one can even think of realistic alternatives. For example, children who avoid school for prolonged periods because of emotional problems sometimes need to reintegrate into the school day gradually. The child may suggest that "I could just go back for gym and art to start with," and the parents might agree but not realize that those classes occur at a different time each day. Thus, this plan may not be feasible unless transportation can be arranged for those varying times of day. Furthermore, school personnel may have different ideas about how reintegration should be organized. In this case, school personnel, parents, the therapist, and the child all need to be involved in the problem solving to ensure that a feasible plan is developed based on accurate information.

Sometimes children think there are no alternatives when there are. For example, a timid child who is told the rule "No talking in class" may think that he or she is not allowed to ask the teacher for help. Conversely, a child raised with few limits may assume choice where there is none. For example, after agreeing to play the clarinet in the school band, a child may ask midway through the term, "Can I switch to the trumpet instead?" and be disappointed when the music teacher refuses.

In this case, reframing the problem as "coping with playing clarinet this year" is helpful. Being clear about what alternatives do or do not exist is important to ensure that problem solving is productive.

AGE-RELATED DIFFERENCES IN ALTERNATIVES

The alternatives children produce do vary somewhat with age. Younger children are more dependent on others than older children; so, they often think of more support-seeking alternatives that need parental involvement than older children do. For example, a younger child might want to make a friend by having a parent arrange a playdate, while an older child might just invite classmates over or go to a movie with them. The parent might still end up paying for the movie, but the child is initiating most of the behaviors needed to build the friendships.

Encourage children to take this kind of initiative as soon as they are able to do so, and to implement their solutions as independently as possible. Problem solving and implementing their own solutions are wonderful ways to build children's confidence and self-esteem. If parental involvement is needed, encourage children to make respectful requests. Sometimes "How to talk to Mom about this" or "How to talk to Dad about this" becomes a separate problem to be solved! If the child really needs your support to implement a solution or to discuss it with his or her parents, provide only as much support as is needed. Children are often able to do more than adults think they can!

Adolescents may solve some problems quite independently. For example, a grade 8 student with a large assignment due the next day may realize quickly that the alternatives include asking the teacher for an extension, doing an all-night study session to complete the work, or accepting a lower grade if the work is only partly done. The alternatives can be evaluated fairly quickly within the same session, and a choice can be made and implemented with only minimal involvement by the therapist or the parents. Parental reaction to the outcome may, of course, prompt the student to do something different the next time, but overall he or she has addressed the issue without much help.

Other teen problems do require some parental involvement, however. For example, older adolescents who can drive may want to use the car to go out with friends but may have difficulty convincing their parents to allow this. "How do I get my parents to trust me with the car?" may be a reasonable problem definition. Alternatives might include: follow other house rules to build parental trust; make a plan for the evening with friends, including how and when the car will be returned; provide the telephone number of the place where the group of friends is going; and/or offer to pay for gas mileage. Ultimately, however, lending the car to the young person is still a parental decision. Resist the temptation to agree to talk to the parents on the adolescent's behalf, even if you think the teen is responsible enough to take the car for the evening. The goal of working with adolescents is to help them solve their problems, not to solve them on their behalf, and few things are as unpleasant for a therapist as being caught in the middle of a family argument.

COMMON CHALLENGES

Children Who Have Difficulty Generating Alternatives

Sometimes children respond to a therapist's attempts to discuss alternative solutions with silence, a shoulder shrug, or "I dunno." There are many potential reasons for this. Some children grow up in authoritarian families where they are rarely asked for their opinions. Children in these families learn that it is important to follow the rules and tell the grown-ups what they want to hear. When asked to generate new solutions or to "brainstorm," these ideas are foreign to them. They may become anxious about not providing the "right" answer. Children who have perfectionist tendencies (regardless of family background) face a similar dilemma. For these children, considerable time may be needed to develop trust and reassure them that you will not criticize or judge their ideas as "right" or "wrong." Show that you are genuinely interested in what the child has to say. If he or she still appears tense, take a playful approach by, for example, setting a goal of five new ideas and drawing a thermometer that is labeled from 1 to 5. Then, challenge the child to make the temperature rise!

Further ideas for prompting, providing, or positively reinforcing alternatives are listed in Table 4.1. Prompts are listed at the top, as it is helpful to get the child to come up with as many ideas as possible before providing any. Children are usually more motivated to pursue their own ideas than the therapist's ideas, and being able to attribute a successful outcome to one's own idea is a real confidence booster. When providing an alternative, ask for the child's opinion. This practice allows the child at least some sense of ownership of the idea and thus also helps with motivation and confidence.

Positive reinforcement may be needed in more challenging cases. Praise every attempt the child makes to participate in the discussion, even

TABLE 4.1. Helping Children Generate Alternatives

Strategy	Examples
Prompting alternatives and/or hypothetical solutions	• "What else could you do?" • "What other possibilities are there?" • "Let's pretend you didn't need to do this. What would you do then?" • "Let's see how many wild ideas we can come up with." • "Say the first thing that comes to mind, even if it seems silly or not possible." • "Let's write down everything you can think of. We can always throw away the paper later if none of it makes sense. And, who knows? Something might." • "What might your friend do?" (Talking about friends is often less threatening than talking about oneself.) • "What might you tell your friend to do?" • "I know you can come up with one more idea. What is it?" (A bit pushy, but sometimes more effective than asking for lots of ideas.)
Providing alternatives (while making sure to ask for the child's opinion so that the child takes ownership of the idea)	• "What would happen if you did this?" • "I wonder if you could do that. What do you think?" • "Could you try this? How would that be for you?" • "Another possibility might be to do that. Should we consider that?" • "If I were in your shoes, I might think about doing this." • "What do you think?" • "Some possibilities might be A, B, or C. Which of those sounds like it might work for you?"
Positive reinforcement of alternatives (regardless of their merit)	• Praise every effort with "What a neat/great/cool idea!" • Offer a reward—for example: "Let's put a sticker on the page [or quarter on the table for a more materialist child] for every idea you can come up with."

if it seems off-topic. Try to make the praise specific to the idea expressed by the child, if possible, to make it more meaningful. For example, if the child suggests reminding himself to make his lunch by taping a picture of a sandwich on the fridge, it is more meaningful to the child if you say "That's a great reminder. It looks tasty too!" instead of just saying "Good idea." If participation is still very limited, try tangible reinforcements like stars or stickers. In addition, ask parents if there is a particular type of positive reinforcement that works well with their child.

Children can also have difficulty generating alternatives if they are depressed, have poor self-esteem, or have struggled unsuccessfully with problems in the past (e.g., children with unrecognized learning disabilities who have repeatedly failed at school). These children may display what has been termed "learned helplessness." This means that they have learned that it makes no difference what they do or say because outcomes are dictated by others or by circumstances. Believing that their efforts will not affect the outcome of a situation, they do not bother to try. For these children, it is important to structure the problem-solving situation so that every effort is rewarded. Sometimes the therapist must offer praise every time the child opens his or her mouth regardless of what is said, even if it is irrelevant, as in the next example.

> KM: Steve, I know your parents want you to enroll in one after-school activity so you can meet some new friends. Are you OK with that?
>
> STEVE: I guess so.
>
> KM: What sort of activity would you enjoy?
>
> STEVE: (*Shrugs.*) I dunno.
>
> KM: Well, let's say you could do anything in the world, even if it sounds fantastic or silly, what would you do?
>
> STEVE: Like I said, I dunno.
>
> KM: Some kids like sports, other kids like martial arts or activities like scouting, other kids like something more creative like music or drama. What sort of kid are you?
>
> STEVE: A pretty dumb one, I guess, 'cause I can't do any of those things.
>
> KM: Wow! That's an important comment, Steve. [positive reinforcement] If you feel that down about yourself, no wonder you're not keen to do an activity right now! What's made you feel that way? Did something happen to you?
>
> STEVE: (*crying*) It's just my parents are always wanting me to be like my straight-A sister, and that's just not me! [Steve's definition of the problem] I wish they would leave me alone!
>
> KM: (*after a pause and some tissues*) What can I do to help? Would you like me to meet with you and your parents so you can tell them how you feel? Would you like to tell them yourself? [offering alternatives for his problem]

STEVE: Maybe we could both meet with them [his selection of an alternative], but I'm not sure it would do any good [a negative comment I can ignore].

KM: I think that's a fine idea. [positive reinforcement of his choice] Let's give it a try.

Rewarding effort will often get a depressed child to talk about something relevant to his or her life. Then one can either redirect the conversation to the problem at hand or, as in Steve's case, redefine the problem in a way that is more helpful to the child.

Finally, children can have cognitive limitations that hamper their ability to generate alternatives. This problem is particularly common among younger children or children with learning difficulties. In this case, one would move quickly down to the section in Table 4.1 on providing alternatives while still asking for the child's opinion. After several rounds of "multiple choice" with alternatives provided by the therapist, some of these children are able to generate their own alternatives. For example, Suzy is a 6-year-old girl who plays well with other children in the schoolyard but doesn't have any close friends.

SUZY: I wish I had a best friend like everyone else.

KM: You already know some kids at school. Maybe one of them could become a closer friend. Would you like that?

SUZY: Yes, that would be nice.

KM: Is there anyone in particular you would like to become better friends with?

SUZY: Sarah. She's always nice, and she likes horses just like me.

KM: So, what could you do to get closer to Sarah?

SUZY: (looking puzzled) I don't know.

KM: Usually, people get closer as they spend more time together. [providing an alternative] How could you spend some more time with Sarah?

SUZY: I don't know. Maybe go to her house? [a nice alternative]

KM: That might be fun! [positive reinforcement] Do you know where she lives?

SUZY: No. Close to the school, I think.

KM: How could you find out?

SUZY: Ask her, I guess. But I don't know if her mom would let me come over.

KM: So, how could you find out if it's OK to come over?

SUZY: I don't know. I never see her mom.

KM: Could you, for example, find out Sarah's phone number so you could talk to her mom, or maybe give her your phone number? Your mom might even know Sarah's number since she lives in the neighborhood. [providing alternatives]

SUZY: Yeah, I think I'll ask my mom.

KM: And if your mom doesn't know?

SUZY: Then I'll ask if I can give Sarah our phone number.

KM: Sounds good. One of those is sure to work! [positive reinforcement] What will you do when Sarah comes over?

SUZY: Let me think … I could show her my horse books and my stuffed animals, we could play my favorite game, or if it's a nice day we could play on my swing set in the yard. [generating alternatives]

KM: Wow! Sarah will be a lucky girl! [positive reinforcement specific to her ideas]

Children Who See Only One Solution

Some children are unwilling to consider alternatives to their preferred solution. Reasons for this can include oppositionality (common in children with diagnoses that include oppositional defiant disorder, ADHD, obsessive–compulsive disorder, or autism spectrum disorders) or previous bad experiences in similar situations. Bad experiences sometimes come to light when one gently challenges the preferred solution, as in the example of Jed.

JED: I don't want to help with the play backstage. I'd rather just pay my ticket and watch.

KM: I thought you liked setting up lights and hooking up the sound system. Your dad said you were really good at that last year.

JED: Yeah, and look what happened! I thought I was supposed to do a spotlight on the two main characters, and I was only supposed to do it on one. Then the second guy thought he was in the dark and started changing, everybody laughed, and he beat the crap out of me after the show. That's what I got for volunteering!

KM: Well, I can see why you don't want a repeat performance of that! Would it have worked out differently if someone had given you clearer instructions upfront?

JED: Sure! I wouldn't have screwed up!

KM: Imagine, for a minute, if that happened and things turned out really well. Would you still want to just buy a ticket? Would you miss out on anything by not helping backstage?

JED: I'd miss being part of the team and feeling like what I did helped the play succeed. But it wouldn't happen, because the stage manager never gives you details ahead of time.

KM: Then the stage manager has a problem. He is asking people to help but not being clear, so he sets them up for failure. It's surprising anyone would want to help with the production!

JED: Actually, he only has one person backstage so far, and that's his son. Nobody else wants to do it.

KM: Oh, dear! That's not good for the play. Do you think he's aware why people are staying away from the job?

JED: No. I guess I could tell him. But I won't agree to do anything until he spells everything out exactly!

KM: If I were the stage manager, I'd think that was a pretty good deal.

JED: OK. I'll see what he says.

In this case, Jed is not really being rigid or oppositional. He has been hurt by an embarrassing and painful experience and fears he cannot go back to a job he enjoys without risking further embarrassing and painful experiences. He's defensive, but ultimately he is able to find a solution that seems consistent with his wishes and that is helpful and safe.

In the case of a child who is truly oppositional, this approach of gently challenging the preferred solution will not work. If Jed were oppositional, the conversation might proceed as follows:

JED: I don't want to help with the play backstage. I'd rather just pay for my ticket and watch.

KM: I thought you liked setting up lights and hooking up the sound system. Your dad said you were really good at that last year.

JED: What does he know? My dad's never worked on a play. He knows nothing.

KM: What about you? Is the lighting and sound system interesting to you, even a little bit? [I challenge one more time, just in case Jed is angry at his father but willing to problem-solve if we don't mention Dad.]

JED: Like I said, I'll pay for my ticket and watch. Case closed.

At this point, I wouldn't persist in what is likely to be a fruitless discussion. Instead, I would either shift to a problem that Jed is more motivated to work on or, if the oppositional attitude is more persistent, stop working individually with Jed and meet with his parents. Parents are sometimes able to shed light on the reasons for their children's behavior, enabling these to be addressed. If they cannot do so, the therapeutic agreement may need to be revisited. Oppositional behaviors usually need consistent management by all the adults in the child's life (parents, school officials, and the therapist), before the child becomes willing to change them. Once such consistent behavior management is in place, the child may be amenable to further problem solving.

Children Who Generate Too Many Alternatives

Some children quickly generate large numbers of alternatives, leaving the therapist feeling rather overwhelmed. Sometimes this occurs when the child is very bright and creative, though extreme worriers (children with generalized anxiety disorder) and children with attention problems can also be prolific producers of alternatives. Worriers typically elaborate on each alternative by thinking about various hypothetical outcomes, sometimes leading to more alternatives. For example, a child worried about preparing for a test might say:

"I could prepare for my test by asking my friend for her notes, because I missed a class when I was sick last week, but then she might want my notes for another subject, and my mother doesn't like me lending out my notes, so I'd have to argue with her, which would put me in a bad mood and make it hard to concentrate when I study, or I could go in early for extra help from my teacher, but I've done that so many times she's probably sick of seeing me, and besides she doesn't explain things very well, so I might not understand any more than I do now (which is not very much), or I could look up some of the stuff online, except the quality of information on the Internet is not always great, and my dad might need to use the computer the same time I need it, or.... "

The therapist would interject, "Hold on a minute. Let's slow down and write down some of those ideas." It's important to interrupt this monologue to limit the alternatives, or the poor child won't have any time to study at all!

By contrast, children with attention problems are likely to include irrelevant tangents among their alternatives and may lose track of the problem altogether. For the same problem (test preparation), an inattentive child might say:

"I should find my notes. I think they're in my locker. Maybe they're not, because my locker's really messy. My teacher keeps telling us to clean our lockers, but who wants to stay late after school for that? Soccer practice started last week. I think our team has a pretty good shot at the title this year. You know, we made it to the semifinals last year. This year we've got a really good goalie. I just hope we don't have to play Birchwood in the first round. They're tough."

The therapist would interject, "Speaking of tough, how are you going to prepare for that test?"

In both examples above, the therapist needs to interrupt the child at some point to redirect him or her to the process of problem solving. Having the worried or creative child write down alternatives will slow the thought process considerably and also enable the therapist to set some reasonable limits on the length of the list. If the child is distressed by the limits, have him or her short-list the top three or four ideas. Encourage the child to prioritize the alternatives that sound most realistic or feasible.

The inattentive child may need to be redirected to the problem several times before any relevant ideas worth writing down emerge. Patiently do so, and then praise and reiterate on-task comments. If the child cannot concentrate well enough to do all the problem-solving steps in one session, take breaks after each step or two. Use concrete visual reminders (for example, a colorful reminder card) to spell out the steps. These props can make it easier to redirect the child and can also facilitate independent use of the steps in children who cannot remember them easily.

When Parents Will Not Consider Certain Alternatives

Sometimes a child will generate alternatives that parents may find objectionable. If the child goes home and tells his or her parents about all of the alternatives discussed in the session, the parents may become alarmed and question your therapeutic skills or even your sanity! It is helpful, at the outset, to inform parents that many ideas will be discussed and evaluated in therapy but few will ever be acted upon. As a therapist, you can also reassure them that you would never encourage or hide from them any of their child's ideas that might be dangerous. Furthermore, helping their child think about different possibilities will, in the long run, promote good judgment and effective life skills.

If parents want to discuss certain choices in light of their cultural norms and values, this is certainly appropriate and may be helpful to the child. For example, it may be helpful to clarify that parents object to a child's participation in a particular sport not because they dislike the sport but rather because practices occur on a day that is set aside for religious observances. In this case, sports participation may still be possible for the child on a different day of the week.

In general, parents often need to be involved at the next problem-solving step (evaluating and selecting an alternative), especially in younger children whose alternatives may depend on parental participation. Asking parents to be patient and wait for that step (which will usually occur in the next session) may be helpful in reducing anxiety about various strange-sounding alternatives.

Finally, try to avoid siding with the child against the parents or vice versa. Parents pay the bills; so, if they feel you are undermining their authority, the child may not be your client for long. On the other hand, children whose parents and therapists side against them feel outnumbered and victimized—hardly a good place to start from when building a therapeutic alliance. Find alternatives (and help the child find alternatives) that respect what is most important to the child and the parents. These "win–win" solutions are more likely to be implemented and to leave the child feeling successful but not alienated from the family.

Clients Who Want You to Give Them the Alternatives

Some people, regardless of age, do not like to take responsibility for their problems. These people expect you to provide the alternatives or expect you to select the best alternative, or both. They are willing to give up their freedom and have you dictate the outcome for the sake of avoiding responsibility. If things go wrong, they are not to blame—you are. If things go well, they will thank you, but they have learned very little in the process, as you did most of the work. They may also recommend you to their friends, who are usually just as unwilling to take responsibility for their problems as they are. Needless to say, I have met several families where the parents had this sort of attitude.

One example of a decision that therapists are sometimes pressured to make is whether or not the child should change schools if the current school environment seems less than ideal. On the surface, it seems very simple: list the schools the child is eligible to attend (the alternatives), and then look at the advantages and disadvantages of each, including the stress/disruption of making a switch from the school the child presently attends. In addition, I sometimes caution families that I am not an educational consultant or expert in the education system, as this is simply not part of psychiatric training in most jurisdictions. Nevertheless, discussions may sound something like this:

KM: So, Jason tells me he may be going to St. Mary's in the fall.

MOTHER: That's what my husband and I wanted to talk to you about. My husband couldn't join us because he's traveling on business; so, I agreed to ask you: Do you think St. Mary's is the best school for Jason? I've heard good things about it, and he really gets picked on by the other kids at St. Bridget's, but I know you said that school switches are not good for anxious children.

KM: Actually, I said that school switches can be stressful for anxious children, as they are for all children. But, if one school is clearly more suitable than another, sometimes a stressful switch is "short-term pain for long-term gain."

MOTHER: Good. So, you think he should go to St. Mary's. My husband thought we should wait a year, but I told him you would agree it was best to switch now.

KM: Hold on a minute, I didn't say he should necessarily go to St. Mary's. Let's look at the advantages and disadvantages of each school.

JASON: Good, 'cause I like the cafeteria food at St. Bridget's, and my friend Joe is staying there too.

KM: OK, Jason. Those are some advantages of St. Bridget's. Now, what are the disadvantages?

MOTHER: (*interrupting*) He's not academically challenged there, doctor, and the boys there are all really rough. St. Mary's has a much better program, and it's a nicer area.

KM: Jason, what do you think?

JASON: I guess I could go to St. Mary's. My dad says we should do whatever you decide.

KM: You're the one who has to live with the decision, Jason, so I think you need to be part of this. Let's make a chart of the advantages and disadvantages of St. Mary's and St. Bridget's, and everyone can contribute ideas. Then, we'll have a better idea of which one makes sense for you, Jason. Mom, do you want to write down the ones you already mentioned?

MOTHER: (*looking at her watch*) I'm not sure we should drag this out. Can't you just tell us the answer, or are there other schools you would recommend?

At this point, I had to resist the urge to scream at Jason's mother. Instead, I decided to patiently tell her that I did not have "the answer" because it would be different for every child and family, depending on the specific factors they valued in a school and the logistics of having Jason make (or not make) a change. Then I set another appointment to talk about the issue with both parents present as well as Jason. Unfortunately, that appointment was never kept. I suppose the family moved on to someone who was willing to give them "the answer."

When the Therapist Is Concerned about Certain Alternatives

Occasionally, a child will propose an alternative that is concerning because it seems ill advised, dangerous, or unethical. In most cases, the alternative can be noted but discussed and then challenged in the next step of the problem-solving plan (the evaluation of alternatives and the selection of the preferred one or ones). If we want children to think and brainstorm freely, we should not be too quick to judge the thoughts they present, or else they will begin to censor themselves rather than disclosing potentially unacceptable thoughts. It is preferable to take the attitude "They're just thoughts. Thoughts can't hurt people. Only actions can do that." In fact, I often spell this out verbatim for children who are reluctant to tell me about certain thoughts. The open discussion of alternatives—even disturbing ones—enables us to learn about our preferences, values, and reasons for making certain choices.

The only situation where I would change this practice is one where I thought the client was considering an alternative that might cause serious self-harm or harm to others. In this case, I would not end the session until that possibility had been ruled out, and I would not necessarily respect confidentiality. All my clients are told at the outset of treatment that confidentiality rules do not apply if I hear about truly dangerous information.

Interestingly, the same threatening comment could result in a very different outcome, depending on the client and the context. Clinical judgment is often needed to distinguish the innocuous from the dangerous. For example, the appropriate response to the comment "I could strangle him" would be different if it occurred in an exchange with a timid and otherwise well-mannered 7-year-old girl than in an exchange with an angry and impulsive teen boy.

SEVEN-YEAR-OLD STACY

KM: I know you're frustrated when your little brother tattles on you to your parents. How could you handle that?

STACY: I could strangle him! I even imagine it sometimes.

KM: Wow! It must be hard when your feelings get out of control like that. [empathizing and reframing the comment as a "feeling" rather than a plan of action] So, let's say you did strangle your little brother. What then?

STACY: Oh, I could never do that! I just get so mad at him! [She confirms my suspicion that this is all about angry feelings, not necessarily a plan of action.]

KM: I know. So, we really need to figure out what you can do when you get mad, right?

STACY: Yeah, I guess so.

Stacy is cooperative and clearly unlikely to inflict any life-threatening injuries on her brother. By acknowledging her feelings, however, I have identified a good problem to focus on in the subsequent discussion. Her parents are probably already aware of the sibling rivalry, so nobody else needs to be involved at this point.

FIFTEEN-YEAR-OLD ROB

KM: We were talking about the guy who embarrassed you in front of your girlfriend. How are you planning to deal with that?

ROB: I could strangle the *@&! He thinks he can get away with this, but no way! Me and my buddies know where he lives. He walks his dog every night, same place, same time. That's the last time he'll diss yours truly—or *anybody*, if you know what I mean.

KM: Rob, you have every right to be angry, but going after the guy with your buddies will just get you into trouble. There must be another way to handle this.

ROB: Never mind. On my street, we have our own way of handling things.

At this point, Rob will not continue the discussion, or entertain any other alternatives. I have no choice but to report his plan to his parents and to his intended victim. If the parents are not sure they can keep Rob away from the other boy, the police also need to be contacted.

Threats of self-harm can also be challenging, as in the case of Stan, age 14.

STAN: Sometimes I think killing myself would be a way out of this mess.

KM: It must seem horrible, but that's a pretty extreme solution. Are there other solutions that you could consider? [empathy and redirection of the problem]

STAN: Maybe, but I'm too tired to think of them right now. I've had it. I want out! (*Puts his head in his hands and sobs—clearly unable to continue with problem solving.*)

KM: It must seem like life is unbearable right now. How seriously have you thought about ending it? [I try to determine whether Stan is temporarily distressed or rather has a deliberate plan to kill himself.]

STAN: Seriously. I keep looking at the train tracks after I leave your office.

KM: Stan, I don't think you're safe leaving here today. You need to be in the hospital.

STAN: OK.

Not all threats of self-harm need to result in hospitalization, but when dealing with depressed teens like Stan with an immediate and feasible suicide plan, it is always better to be safe than sorry. Note that if Stan had come up with other alternatives to his problem we could have evaluated those in the next problem-solving step. However, he should definitely not leave the office until the alternative of suicide has been fully investigated to make sure he is safe. There are numerous resources on more thorough evaluation of suicide risk in children and teens (see, e.g., Berman, Jobes, & Silverman, 2005).

When There Really Is No Alternative

Sometimes people hope that problem solving will result in a logical and pleasant outcome to any situation for themselves and their children. This is simply not true. There are situations where our ability to control the outcome is limited or nonexistent, no matter how many creative ideas we put on the table. When a tooth is broken, we must go to the dentist to have it fixed or suffer serious consequences to our health. When a pet dies, we must mourn and let go. Pretending that we have choices in these situations is foolish. We do not—we must simply endure them.

Children, too, must endure difficult situations sometimes. As therapists, our role at such times is not to problem-solve but to listen to them, to share in the desperation and helplessness they feel without letting it overwhelm us, and to support whatever ability they have to understand the situation and to get through it. Even young children can understand that we cannot choose our circumstances but we can choose how to respond to them. Facing the dentist with courage (or even just facing the dentist) or finding a way to commemorate a beloved pet (or even just saying good-bye) may not be "preferred solutions," but they are important experiences that are a part of growing up. Situations that cannot be changed may not be amenable to problem solving, but we can still help our young clients to cope with them calmly and effectively.

CHOICE WITHIN LIMITS

When alternatives are provided that are designed to influence choice in a particular direction, some people consider this behavior modification rather than problem solving. Nevertheless, it is worth explaining, as most parents use this approach at least occasionally with their children, and it can be a useful starting point for problem solving when children are not used to generating their own alternatives yet. What is meant by "choice within limits"? Basically, the child is told, "You could do *this* or *that*. Which one makes sense to you?" The alternatives, however, are designed so that both follow the same underlying rule. For example:

IN A PRESCHOOLER

"You could eat broccoli or cauliflower with your dinner. Which one would you like?" (Underlying rule: you are eating a vegetable with dinner.)

IN A YOUNG TEEN

"If you want to do a sleepover with your friend, I can drive you there if you tell me by 7 P.M. You could also decide later, but then you would have to arrange for your friend's mother to drive. Which would you prefer?" (Underlying rule: I don't drive you places after 7 P.M.)

The main advantages of choice within limits are that it is simple, quick, and often more readily accepted by children than a strict rule. The main disadvantages are that children eventually figure out (and may resent) that they are being told they have a choice when instead a rule is being enforced, and that, as well, children learn very little as a result of choices within limits. They learn little because this approach does not allow rules to be broken or mistakes to be made. The process is carefully staged by adults; so, children obtain guidance but cannot learn from their mistakes. Most of us learn more effectively from life experience than from advice; so, choice within limits is not a very effective teaching tool.

Chapter 5

Step 3: Evaluating Alternatives and Making a Choice

HUMAN DECISION-MAKING BEHAVIOR

Once the client has generated a number of alternatives, selecting one seems relatively straightforward. Most people have, at some point in their lives, made a list of pros and cons for various choices and then made a decision. Of course, children have a more limited range of choices, given their relatively less powerful position in society. They must also rely on their parents' judgment as to what is or is not an acceptable choice for them to make at a given age. Most parents, however, will allow their children a gradually increasing range of choices as they mature and demonstrate increasingly responsible behavior. Conversely, gaining practice at making choices through problem solving can contribute to the child's ability to behave independently and become more responsible. Programs designed to foster resilience in children often use problem solving for this reason (Brooks & Goldstein, 2001).

Before describing the process of encouraging effective decision making in children, however, it is worth reviewing some of what is known about human decision-making behavior more generally. Factors that can influence decision making include: speed (impulsive vs. reflective decision making), temporal perspective (short-term vs. long-term gains), individual values (e.g., preference for novelty vs. "tried-and-true" alternatives; preference for socially desirable vs. idiosyncratic choices), the feasibility of various alternatives, and the influence of others (e.g., the therapist, parents, or peers). These will now briefly be described. In children, the developmental level can interact with any of these factors to further influence decision making.

Problem solving steps generally result in reflective decision making, making them particularly helpful for children who are prone to impulsivity (Kendall, 1992), for example, those with ADHD. Studies suggest that adults experienced in a particular occupational field tend to use more reflective decision making than those who are inexperienced (Wainwright, Shepard, Harman, & Stephens, 2010) and that reflective decision making requires use of the prefrontal areas of the brain (Yarkoni, Braver, Gray, & Green, 2005). These areas of the brain continue to develop well into young adulthood. Given their youth and inexperience, children and adolescents are generally more prone to impulsive decision making than adults are. For the most part, reflective decision-making is thought to result in better decisions because it minimizes the risk of impulsively choosing an alternative that later turns out to be suboptimal. Excessive reflection can be very time-consuming, though, and sometimes can prevent a person from ever making a decision. This problem can occur in people who doubt their own decision making ability, and is also common in people with obsessive–compulsive disorder.

"Temporal perspective" refers to people's ability to perceive and value solutions that result in long-term benefits, even if they are not immediately appealing in the short term. For example, having a glass of water instead of an ice cream cone on a hot day may seem unappealing, but it will avoid weight gain in the long run. Most people, however, place a high value on immediate reward and tend to behave accordingly (Luhmann, 2009). Kable and Glimcher (2010), for example, found that the subjective value people attribute to a temporally distant alternative declines exponentially in relation to the soonest available reward. People experienced in a given field tend to have a longer temporal perspective than people less experienced in the same field. For example, clinicians tend to value treatment suitability (likely to result in successful treatment in the long run) more than the urgency of a referral, but the reverse is true for health care officials and lay people (Fredelius, Sandell, & Lindqvist, 2002). Children's temporal perspective is shorter than that of adults. Given their youth, inexperience, and short temporal perspective, children are prone to choosing immediately gratifying alternatives.

The value people place on various alternatives can depend on a host of factors, including cultural background, social influences, temperament (e.g., a novelty-seeking temperament vs. a risk-averse temperament), and current circumstances. Individuals of all ages often prefer solutions that mimic others' behavior (Watanabe, 2009), speaking to the importance of social influences. Emotions seem to mediate the relationship between circumstances and values. Thus, people are more likely to choose novel alternatives when emotionally distressed (Schweickhardt, Leta, & Bauer, 2005), consistent with the common adage that a crisis represents an opportunity for change. Once a decision is made, however, people tend to place a higher value on the alternative chosen than they did before the decision was made (Svenson & Jakobsson, 2010), as if needing to convince themselves that they made the right choice.

Examining the feasibility of various alternatives is particularly important in young children (e.g., preschoolers), who often engage in wishful or even magical thinking, owing to their cognitive immaturity. Younger children are also more susceptible to family influences when making decisions than older children are. Conversely, peer or media influences are sometimes overvalued by adolescents. Internet marketing strategies have been particularly successful with this age group (Lin & Wang, 2008), underscoring the importance of encouraging a healthy skepticism of media messages when working with this age group. Finally, therapists have a role in guiding client decisions at all ages, if only to help their clients avoid choices that are clearly harmful. Therapist influence may be limited, though, as people who use consultants to help with decision making often strengthen their resolve to do what they originally planned (Bowers & Pipes, 2000).

In summary, decision making should ideally be reflective (but not excessively so), should utilize long as well as short temporal perspectives, be sensitive to the client's circumstances and values, and result in a feasible and safe solution to the problem. Informed by these facts, we can now examine how to help children select among various alternatives when they are problem solving. Questions that help in prompting children's decision-making behaviors are listed in Table 5.1, and each behavior is discussed below. Therapists can refer to this list to elicit particular behaviors, but they would be unlikely to use all of these questions in the same problem-solving exercise.

HELPING CHILDREN TO BE
APPROPRIATELY REFLECTIVE

To encourage reflective decision making, the therapist must prevent the child from choosing impulsively and then guide him or her through

TABLE 5.1. Helping Children Select Alternatives

Decision-making behavior	Questions to prompt that behavior
Using reflection	• "What would be good about that choice? Anything else?" • "What would *not* be good about that choice? Anything else?" • "Do you need to know more about that choice? What do you need to know? How can you find the answer?"
Using temporal perspective	• "How would you feel right after doing that?" • "How would you feel a week/a month/a year later?" • "How would you feel in the long run?" • "What would happen right after you did that?" • "What would happen a week/a month/a year later?" • "What would happen in the long run?"
Considering circumstances	• "Could you do that on your own?" • "Who would need to help? Do you think they would help?" • "Would anything else need to change in order for this to work?"
Considering personal values	• "What choice allows you to do/get what is most important to you? What makes it so important?" • "Would you be comfortable with that choice? Why?" • "What is your favorite thing in the world to do?"
Ensuring safety	• "Are there any risks to doing this?" • "How could you make sure nobody gets hurt?"
Ensuring feasibility	• "Do you think this idea will work? Why?" • "Is that really possible?" • "Would anything stop you from doing this?" • "Would you need anyone's help or any money to do this?"

the decision step by step. Gently redirect the impulsive child by saying, "Let's take a minute to think this through" or something similar. Then encourage the child to examine the advantages and disadvantages for each alternative that could be chosen. If more information is needed about one or more alternatives, help the child find that information and record it. Writing things down further slows the decision-making process to ensure that it is reflective and also provides a visual reminder of what has been discussed. When the advantages and disadvantages for each alternative are clear, encourage the child to look them over, select an alternative, and justify the choice.

Some children will do a tally of advantages, disadvantages, or calculate the difference between the two for each alternative, hoping for a mathematical formula for making decisions. This is usually not helpful, as one particular advantage or disadvantage may be more important to the child than the others. A good alternative doesn't necessarily have the most advantages, but it should address whatever the child considers most important about the situation.

For example, a young teen was asked by her classmates to lead the environment club at school. She was uncertain whether or not to accept this role because there had not been an election for the position and she had very little leadership experience. However, she did not want to offend her classmates by turning them down. She debated the decision for several days. Finally, her therapist asked her what was most important to her about the situation. "That the environment club raises the school's awareness about environmental issues this year," she replied without hesitation. Since there was no other obvious leader for the club and she had this clear goal, she decided to accept the job pending a vote by her peers. She was elected and became a confident and competent leader at her school.

Conversely, it may be possible to rule out some alternatives fairly quickly because they are clearly not in the child's best interest even though there may appear to be some advantages to them. For example, having a tantrum in class on the day the child is expected to take a test has the advantage of allowing the child to avoid the test. Unfortunately, it will also result in some very detrimental consequences for the child, so it should probably be ruled out as an alternative.

What about the child who rushes into impulsive choices repeatedly? As mentioned, children with ADHD sometimes have difficulty avoiding impulsive choices since impulsivity is a hallmark of the disorder. Other children may behave impulsively in certain situations. For example, a child may be tired of thinking about a problem in detail and may want a break. Rather than asking for a break, he or she may rush through the task by choosing the first thing that comes to mind. Another possibility is that the child is not really interested in the problem being discussed. Perhaps it is an issue that matters to his parents but not to the child himself. He may want to get through the task quickly to get his parents to stop dwelling on the problem rather than being genuinely interested in finding the best solution. Disliking the therapist or therapy sessions can also result in decreased interest in the problem and consequently making an impulsive choice. Explore these possibilities if the child seems unwilling or unable to slow down in response to the "Using reflection" questions in the table.

What about the child who is overly reflective and generates lengthy lists of advantages and disadvantages without coming to a decision? There can be several reasons for this behavior. Depressed children and teens can be prone to rumination and may doubt their own abilities to make decisions. Anxious children may fear trying a new behavior and engage in lengthy deliberations with the therapist in order to avoid change. Perfectionist children may have difficulty because there appears to be no perfect choice, since almost all alternatives have at least one disadvantage. Some children also have a strong fear of making a choice that meets with adult disapproval or criticism. Explore these possibilities if the child seems unwilling or unable to settle on a choice despite your best efforts to help him or her to do so.

To help the child move on, the therapist may have to encourage writing down only the most important advantages or disadvantages, or moving on to the next alternative after a period of time. Sometimes setting a time limit for the task can be helpful, so long as the child does not find this too distressing. Reframing all choices as learning opportunities may also help. In other words, the child's goal should be to try something new and learn from it, even if several tries are needed to find the best solution. Reassure the child that everyone makes "wrong" choices sometimes, and, as long as people learn from their mistakes, this need not be disastrous.

Some children ask many questions about the alternatives or want to seek out large amounts of information about them. Usually this behavior is caused by a fear of being unprepared for the situation and a desire to make it more predictable. If the resulting delay is prolonged, the therapist may need to set limits on this quest for information as well. Reassure the child that a degree of uncertainty about the outcome is inevitable, as none of us can predict the future precisely. Praise the child for tolerating this uncertainty and having the courage to make a choice in spite of it.

HELPING CHILDREN TO USE
TEMPORAL PERSPECTIVE

We have all heard the saying "short-term pain for long-term gain." In many situations, a long-term temporal perspective is helpful. Children who are young or impulsive, however, often seek immediate gratification. When examining alternatives, therapists may need to prompt these children to examine the long-term as well as short-term consequences of each alternative. Some helpful questions to prompt one's temporal perspective are listed in Table 5.1. Depending on the child's personality, the therapist may choose to place more emphasis on either concrete consequences (i.e., what would happen) or consequences for the child's feelings.

Sometimes children can understand that there is a benefit to waiting for something good. For example, waiting for Christmas morning for their gifts ensures that these are a nice surprise that is shared with the whole family. Searching through the cupboards to find their gifts ahead of time may satisfy children's curiosity, but it usually results in a less surprising and therefore less joyful Christmas experience. In other situations, the benefit of waiting is less obvious. Many parents have argued, "You'll enjoy the party more if you finish your homework first." Only very conscientious children are convinced by this argument. Let's look at a situation where a therapist uses temporal perspective in problem solving with a young boy, Timmy.

TIMMY: I want to go out with my friends Saturday, but my dad wants me to do stupid homework!

KM: How could you handle that situation?

TIMMY: I could tell him that all the other parents are letting their kids go.

KM: Do you think he would listen to that idea?

TIMMY: Probably not. The last time I said that he asked if I'd jump off a cliff if all my friends did!

KM: So what else could you do?

TIMMY: I could lie and tell him I have no homework.

KM: How would you feel after doing that?

TIMMY: Fine, because he would let me go and I could enjoy myself.

KM: That might be true on Saturday, but what would happen between you and your dad after that, I mean in the long run?

TIMMY: My dad might find out.

KM: What would happen if he found out?

TIMMY: He would get really mad.

KM: And in the long run?

TIMMY: He wouldn't trust me anymore, so he probably wouldn't let me go out with my friends again for quite a while.

KM: Is there another solution that would work out better in the long run?

TIMMY: Maybe I could make a deal with my dad to get some of the homework done before I go out, and then finish the rest on Sunday.

KM: How do you think he'd react to that plan?

TIMMY: He might be surprised ... I don't usually think ahead that far. But I guess it's worth a try.

I agreed with Timmy, and, at his request, he presented the plan to his father at the end of the appointment. His father agreed, and Timmy stuck to his plan.

So far, I have emphasized the benefits of taking a long-term perspective on decisions, as most children have a relatively short temporal perspective. Some children, however, are overly focused on long-term future outcomes that might arise because of their decisions. This problem is common in anxious children. Anxious children may, for example, avoid going to the movies or going to the ballgame in order to save every penny for college. They might also argue against a spontaneous trip to the beach on a hot day, believing they need every moment to prepare for an upcoming test or examination. For these children, the therapist may wish to highlight the short-term benefits of some decisions and the value of flexibly "going with the flow" of life sometimes. Occasional deviations from one's plan or routine can be fun, and the result is not always disastrous. Successful inventors, for example, sometimes take a playful attitude toward their work. Flexibility is also a helpful attribute when working with others in groups, where children who rigidly cling to their plans are sometimes seen as being obstinate or being poor team players. Flexibility also allows children to better tolerate the inevitable changes in routine they sometimes encounter, such as, for example, having a substitute teacher at school.

HELPING CHILDREN
TO CONSIDER THE CIRCUMSTANCES

Children sometimes assume that they can make choices about matters that are really outside of their control, or conversely that they have no choice about matters over which they can exert some influence or control. When helping children make decisions, it is important to provide a realistic perspective on the extent to which they can influence their circumstances. Erika, for example, had been avoiding school following a flu-like illness and was discussing how she planned to return.

KM: How do you imagine going back to school next week?

ERIKA: My dad will drive me, and I'll meet my best friend, Jade, at school just before the bell. She'll be really happy to see me. Then we'll go to class together, and I'll ask the teacher for the work I missed.

KM: Has your dad agreed to drive you? I thought you usually took the bus.

ERIKA: I don't want the kids on the bus asking me where I've been and looking at me funny. It's better if I get a ride.

KM: I agree it would be more comfortable for you, but has your dad agreed?

ERIKA: He'll probably say he has to go to work, but I think mom will make him drive me.

KM: Let's check that out with your parents. Then we can talk about what to say to the other kids if they ask where you've been. You might run into that question at school even if you don't take the bus.

In this case, Erika is imagining a very positive experience when she returns to school. This suggests that she is motivated to go back, which is encouraging. However, she may be overestimating the control she has over the situation. If her father does not agree to drive her, or her friend Jade does not happen to be waiting for her in the schoolyard, or some children in the schoolyard ask her where she has been, Erika will face a more challenging situation than she expects. As her therapist, I would rather help her prepare for potentially challenging circumstances than assume that everything will work out as well as she anticipates.

Children can also underestimate their ability to influence a situation. Kevin, for example, was a boy who was not very self-confident and whose father wanted him to try out for a competitive soccer team.

KM: I heard that your dad is taking you to the soccer tryouts on Friday. Sounds great! I know that's your favorite sport.

KEVIN: I wish I didn't have to go. I like playing house league at

school, but I don't think I'm good enough for the city league.
Everyone will probably laugh at me.

KM: That's quite a worry. What could you do about this situation?

KEVIN: Nothing. My dad will call me a quitter if I don't go, and I'll
feel totally embarrassed if I do.

KM: What you're really saying, though, is that you could either talk
about the issue with your dad or you could go and participate
in the tryout. That sounds like a choice to me. What would
happen if you did each of those things?

KEVIN: Like I said, if I talked to my dad, he would push me to go.

KM: Does your dad understand the difference in the level of play in
this league versus your house league?

KEVIN: I don't know.

KM: It might be worth explaining that. I don't think he would want
to set you up to fail. If he knows it's a tough league, maybe he
could give you some pointers, or maybe he'd be OK if you tried
out next year.

KEVIN: I don't think he'd listen to me.

KM: Would he listen to someone else who knows about soccer?

KEVIN: Coach Johnson at school, I guess. Maybe I'll ask him to talk
to my dad.

In this case, a few prompts on my part enable Kevin to see that
he does have more influence over the outcome of this situation than he
originally thought. After his coach discussed the soccer tryouts with his
father, his father responded, "So, that's why you were so glum, Kevin! I
was wondering what was wrong. You're a bit young for the city league
this year anyway. I just thought you'd like to gain some experience trying out. Your cousin's going too, and he doesn't have nearly your skills."
When Kevin heard that there would other inexperienced players trying
out, he was no longer worried about embarrassment and decided to go
to the tryouts "just for the experience."

In both examples, adults outside the therapeutic relationship had
to be involved in the decision. This is not unusual. Because children
are relatively powerless as compared to adults, the degree of influence
or control they have over their circumstances often depends upon the
adults in their lives. Children who are able to enlist the help of adults
therefore often have more influence or control than those who cannot. Thus, helping children adapt to their circumstances often involves

improving their ability to relate successfully to important adults in their lives.

Most parents are pleased to see their child trying to solve problems independently, but some parents find this concerning. They secretly hope that the therapist will only allow their child to make the best choice in a given situation and never allow him or her to make a "bad" decision. For example, if Kevin's father had been less understanding, he might have become angry that Kevin was allowed to pursue the option of *not* attending the tryout. In this case, I would have met with Kevin's father separately and discussed the merits of learning from experience. That is, as long as an option is safe, a child can discover its merits from trial and error. Lessons learned from positive and negative experiences are typically remembered better than those learned from books or discussions. Thus, in the long run, children who are allowed to learn from experience typically become more competent and confident than those who are not given this opportunity.

HELPING CHILDREN TO CONSIDER THEIR PERSONAL VALUES

As noted above, the best decision is usually the one that enables the child to get what is most important to him or her, even if that choice does not have the most advantages or the fewest disadvantages on paper. What is most important varies, however, depending on the child's age, temperament, and circumstances. For example, a young child may value time spent playing a game with a parent, while a teen may value an extra hour to stay out with friends. Some children have a strong need for novelty or sensory stimulation. For a thrill-seeker like this, a chance to go down a zipline might be valued more than a school activity. Other children gravitate toward quiet, predictable pursuits. They might feel more comfortable playing chess than ziplining. Some children have a strong need for social acceptance and value choices that seem acceptable in their social circle. Others are rebellious or pride themselves in "marching to their own drummer." Given this variability in what children value, adults should not assume that they always know what children prefer. Consider the following interaction between Max and his mother.

MAX: I don't want to go to gym Wednesday nights any more. I'm too busy. I need some free time.

MOTHER: Too busy? You hardly have any afterschool activities!

What are you going to do—be a couch potato and watch TV all evening?

MAX: No. I just want to unwind after school. I was hoping I could relax and maybe ... play a board game with you. There are lots in my room that we haven't played in ages. Will you have time for that?

MOTHER: I'll need to clean up and do the dishes first, but if you help me with that we will have some time.

MAX: Great! I'll help and then we can play.

Notice that Max's mother assumes he wants to sit on the couch and watch television, but he really values time spent interacting with her. Once she realizes what really matters to Max, she is able to adapt her routine (and his) so he can have it. Therapists should also be wary of assuming they know what children value. See the "Considering personal values" section in Table 5.1 for ways to prompt discussion of what the child values most or is most comfortable with.

Family circumstances can also affect what children value. Thus, children in affluent but busy families may have lots of toys and treats but little time with other family members; so, they may value the latter more. The opposite may be true for children in impoverished families. Abraham Maslow once described a hierarchy of human needs and values that is sometimes helpful to consider when looking at the child's circumstances (Maslow, 1954). He suggested that when basic survival needs (food, shelter, etc.) are met, people focus more on security. When security needs are met, they focus in turn on love or a sense of belonging with other human beings, then sources of self-esteem, and finally what he termed "self-actualization." Self-actualization is the desire to realize one's full potential or "to become more and more what one is, to become everything that one is capable of becoming" (Maslow, 1954, p. 203).

How do Maslow's ideas relate to children's choices? For some children, choices that enable them to feel close to others or that boost their self-esteem are valued more than material rewards. If these children are having difficulty deciding between alternatives, suggest some advantages that have to do with relating to others or taking pride in their abilities, and see how they respond. For other children, the question "What is your favorite thing in the world to do?" elicits sources of self-actualization. The best answer I've ever heard to that question came from an 11-year-old girl who replied, "My favorite thing in the world to do is figure skate. I sail across the ice, and nothing else matters. I have no worries. I only think about what I'm doing, and I feel great." There was no doubt about what mattered most to this girl.

INSISTING THAT CHILDREN CHOOSE SAFE ALTERNATIVES

As therapists, we have a responsibility not only to help children choose safe alternatives but to insist upon them. Most people providing mental health services to children are aware of the need to refer children with suicidal or homicidal ideation to emergency services and to report even a suspicion of child abuse to local authorities. Situations where the child displays poor judgment that might endanger his safety or the safety of those around him can, however, be challenging. Consider the case of Joe, a boy in his teens with fetal alcohol syndrome (known to severely impair social judgment).

> KM: What are your plans for the weekend, Joe?
>
> JOE: I'm gonna go to Club Zero with my buddy Sam. We'll get some E, and pick up a couple of chicks. Good times, man, good times! [Note that Joe freely and rather loudly confesses his plans to use illicit drugs even though his mother is sitting in my waiting room.]
>
> KM: Wasn't that the club you went to last month, when you got arrested?
>
> JOE: Yeah, busted! Man, those cops were nasty. Police brutality! I could sue them, you know.
>
> KM: Still, do you really want to risk going through that again?
>
> JOE: There won't be no cops this time. Sam knows the owner. He made sure.
>
> KM: I'm not sure the cops always tell the owner when they're planning to raid the club. Do you really want to risk another night in jail?
>
> JOE: Well, what else am I gonna do on Saturday? Hang out with my mom's lame friends?
>
> KM: I'm sure there are some fun things to do around town that won't get you arrested, Joe. Let's take a look at the paper and see.

JOE: No way! Sam's gonna expect me to come to the club! He's picking me up.

KM: Does your mother know about this plan?

JOE: She won't stop me. She's five-foot nothing. What's she gonna do?

KM: I don't know, Joe. But I think she has a right to know the kind of stuff you and Sam get into sometimes. You might not like this, but I'm gonna have to tell her. It sounds like you might get into more trouble otherwise.

Joe was not happy that I talked to his mother, and he left the office angry. After a few more repetitions of this scenario, however, he realized that the limits his mother and I set on his behavior were well intentioned and he accepted them. Eventually, we located a youth drop-in center not far from where he lived, where Joe could spend his Saturdays safely and still have fun.

There are other risks teens sometimes take, even if their judgment seems intact most of the time. We have all heard the expression "Maybe it happened to them, but it can't happen to me." This expression is typical of teen thinking. In other words, even when they appreciate the risks, teens sometimes think they are personally invincible. Driving under the influence of alcohol or drugs and risky sexual behavior are common examples of unsafe decisions teens sometimes make.

When discussing these issues with teens, ask leading questions to get them to evaluate the risks themselves whenever possible. Ask questions like "Are there any risks to doing this?" or "How could you make sure nobody gets hurt?" This approach respects teens' ability to think independently and strengthens the reflective thinking needed to make sound and safe decisions. If, as in Joe's case, the teen cannot reflect upon the risks and continues to advocate an unsafe choice, involve the adult(s) responsible for the teen to ensure safety.

Safety concerns can also arise when working with younger children, although these are less common than when working with teens because the child's parents usually ensure safety. Occasionally, however, children will overestimate their abilities or behave impulsively, with tragic consequences. For example, children sometimes drown in pools or lakes because they assume they are safe in the water after a few swimming lessons. Impulsive children sometimes hurt others inadvertently if they, for example, jump off playground equipment without looking ahead to where they will be landing. They can hurt themselves if they engage in a sport and forget to don safety equipment (e.g., forgetting to wear a bicycle helmet). Most of these accidents cannot be averted through problem solving, because they are sudden, unplanned events. However, if a therapist hears about potentially risky situations such as a nonswimmer vacationing at the beach or an impulsive child participating in an unstructured, minimally supervised play activity, it is worth alerting the adults in the child's life to the potential dangers.

HELPING CHILDREN
TO CHOOSE FEASIBLE ALTERNATIVES

Because problem solving encourages learning from experience, people sometimes assume that the client should be allowed to try out any alternative that is safe, no matter how unrealistic it may be. This approach can be harmful, though, in that children who repeatedly try out unrealistic and therefore unsuccessful alternatives can become discouraged and give up on problem solving altogether. Also, children can benefit from learning to anticipate likely outcomes ahead of time. Evaluating the feasibility of an alternative before it is chosen allows for this kind of learning and can therefore often help the child avoid disappointment and discouragement.

Young children may believe that there are magical solutions to their problems. For example, a young child who has been criticized by a teacher might suggest "I will wish for the teacher to disappear" as a possible solution to the problem. The therapist may need to gently remind the child that this is an unlikely outcome and encourage thinking about other more likely solutions.

Older children can also think of solutions that are unlikely to be feasible, but usually these are not magical. Rather, the child may have an idea that is possible only if certain resources (time, money, parental approval, etc.) are available. For example, a child may be worried about missing her mother when she goes away to a conference and propose accompanying her mother on the trip. Her mother, however, may not be able to afford to take her daughter along and may not be able to arrange for someone to babysit the girl while she attends the conference meetings. Another child may want to do an after-school karate program across town but not realize that a parent is not available to drive him there at that time. Working with limited resources is a skill that all of us must learn as we grow up, so it is well worth discussing these issues with children when we help them select a course of action.

Some questions that can prompt children to think about the feasibility of their proposed solutions are listed in Table 5.1. Most children understand that an idea is or is not feasible if prompted to think about it. A few will deny that it is unlikely to work or will insist on trying it even if it is unlikely to work. In this case, accept the fact that experience is a better teacher than you will ever be. Allow these children to try out their proposed solutions, and resist the urge to say "I told you so" the following week. Instead, empathize with their disappointment and see what can be learned from the experience.

Finally, accept that we therapists don't know everything about children's lives. Some children are able to achieve more than we think they can. A 12-year-old girl on the autistic spectrum who announces, "I am going to fly across the country by myself for my 16th birthday" may elicit snickers or pity from adults. Given the focused, single-minded determination of children with this diagnosis, however, she just might do it! Big dreams shouldn't be discouraged. Instead, help the child break the dream down into small realistic steps that are necessary to achieve it. Several discussions with parents and aviation instructors, flying lessons, an air cadet program to allow lots of practice, a chance to "solo," and access to a plane for her "sweet 16" birthday celebration were some of the steps this girl needed to make her dream a reality.

Ultimately, we need to gather information and use our judgment as therapists and as sensible adults to help children decide what is or is not feasible. Similarly, we need some judgment to decide when there has been enough reflection and discussion of temporal perspectives, circumstances, values, and safety. Some decisions can be made in a heartbeat, while others require several discussions. Knowing one's own preferred decision-making style can be helpful in deciding when "enough is enough." If you tend to be impulsive, try to increase the number of questions you ask when helping children select alternatives. If you tend to deliberate about things excessively, try to limit the questions once the child seems comfortable with the decision. Then, get ready for the next step: encouraging the child to try it out!

Chapter 6

Step 4: Trying a New Solution

Thinking about a new solution is often easier than actually putting it into practice. As anyone who has ever tried to keep a New Year's resolution will tell you, old habits die hard. For most people, it takes several weeks to establish a new behavior and sometimes longer. In this chapter, I examine how to increase the chances that children will try out their new solutions, and how to continue encouraging them if they don't do what they planned right away. A checklist for preparing children to try out new solutions is presented in Figure 6.1. Defining the problem, generating alternative solutions, and selecting the best alternative have been discussed in previous chapters. Other aspects of preparation will now be discussed in turn.

MOTIVATION

The new solution, since it was selected from among several alternatives, should be one the child sees as most advantageous. Nevertheless, the child may need your help to be motivated to actually *try* the new solution. It may be worth acknowledging to the child that any change—no matter how advantageous—can be hard. Normalize the struggle to do something different so that the child feels free to talk about any doubts regarding the new solution. "This might not feel natural at first," or

Check if done	Prepare by ...
	Helping the child define a clear situation-specific problem.
	Helping the child examine all reasonable alternatives.
	Helping the child thoughtfully select a safe, feasible solution.
	Ensuring the child is motivated to try the new solution.
	Helping the child try out the new solution in the office, if possible.
	Having the child summarize the plan for implementing the new solution in the real world.
	Having the child specify the day, time, and place for implementation.
	Anticipating possible difficulties with implementation.
	Having a contingency plan if needed.
	Enlisting parental support if needed.
	Encouraging the child to self-reinforce him- or herself for trying the solution.
	Encouraging parental reinforcement if needed.

FIGURE 6.1. A checklist for trying out new solutions.

"You might not feel up to it every day," or "Most kids would find this a bit challenging" are some common statements that normalize the difficulty in making a change. Notice, however, that the statements acknowledge *some* difficulty rather than *a lot of* difficulty. If change is described as being extremely difficult, the child's confidence will be undermined, and so extreme descriptions should be avoided.

If the child looks worried or doubtful when discussing the new solution, ask, "How confident are you that this will work?" If the child is not confident, explore what obstacles he or she anticipates in implementing the new solution and help the child address these obstacles. If the child says, "I'm fine. I know I can do it," be supportive of the child's determined attitude, even if his or her body language indicates some doubt.

Review the questions regarding readiness for change that were discussed early in Chapter 2. Some of these questions may be worth revisiting. Additional questions that can build motivation to try a specific solution include:

- "How will your life/your child's life be different if this solution works?"
- "How will you/your child feel if this works?"

- "How will people important to you/your child react if this works?"
- "What will be missed if this solution is never tried?"
- "What would be a small sign that this solution is starting to work?" (Small signs of progress encourage perseverance.)
- "Can you/your child visualize the new solution and its positive consequences?" (If "yes," the therapist should encourage such visualization. Imagined success is often a powerful motivator toward real success!)

Let's examine the role of motivation for Ben, in his first year of high school, who has decided to try out for the diving team in order to feel that he "belongs."

KM: So, when are the tryouts, Ben?

BEN: (*tentatively*) The day after tomorrow.

KM: You look worried.

BEN: I met some of the guys who are already on the team. Most of them are a foot taller than me!

KM: Well, then, it's natural that you would feel a bit intimidated. Your gymnastics background should help, though. Not every kid has that. Are you still planning to go out?

BEN: I guess so.

KM: Are you sure?

BEN: Well, it seemed like a good idea when we talked about it last week, but now that it's getting closer I'm not so sure.

KM: Let's think about it one more time. What do you predict will happen if you go out and make the team, if you go out and don't make the team, or if you choose not to go out? How would you feel in each situation, and how would people react?

BEN: If I went out and made it, I would feel fantastic! I would tell all my friends, and I would probably make lots of new friends on the team. If I didn't make it, I would be disappointed and maybe embarrassed if I really screwed up a dive. People would understand, though, since it's only my first year at the school. They'd probably tell me to try again next year. If I didn't go out, nobody would care, but I would feel like I chickened out because of all those bigger guys on the team. Plus, I wouldn't know if I could have made it if I tried.

KM: So, what's it going to be?

BEN: I guess I'll give it a try. What have I got to lose?

KM: Sounds like a plan. Let me know how it goes.

Note that Ben is a bright, reflective teen; so, I knew that with a bit of prompting he would understand the consequences of his decision. Younger or less sophisticated children may need more guidance from the therapist to evaluate their decisions.

TESTING THE WATERS

Some new solutions can be tried in the therapist's office before implementing them in the real world. For example, children with phobias of certain animals (spiders, dogs, etc.) are often exposed to those animals in the safety and comfort of the therapist's office before facing them in day-to-day situations. Having an environment where safety is guaranteed and there is a supportive adult present to offer reassurance and guidance makes the exposure easier to tolerate. Similarly, children who rush through their homework, are distracted when doing it, or are unable to start it owing to a fear of mistakes can practice alternative homework strategies with their therapists before using these independently at home. Children can also role-play conversations with their therapists, enabling them to practice new types of interactions with peers, parents, or teachers without any adverse consequences.

Anything that can be simulated in the office is worth trying there first, because most children find new solutions easier to implement in a supportive environment with a supportive adult. Sometimes, especially with younger children, parents or teachers need to provide continued support when the child tries the new solution outside the office. Practicing in the office builds confidence and also helps the child and therapist anticipate difficulties that might arise when implementing the solution outside of the office.

Of course, not all new solutions can be simulated in the therapist's office. Taking the bus independently, for example, can only be partially simulated. The child and therapist can look at the bus route and the bus schedule, plan the walk from the child's home to the bus stop, figure out the correct fare to give the bus driver, and locate the stop where the child must get off the bus. The actual bus ride, however, is only possible outside the office.

AN IMPLEMENTATION PLAN

When the child seems ready to try the new solution outside the office, it is worth reviewing briefly what exactly will be done. Have the child summarize the plan for implementing the new solution, including what he or she plans to do on what day, at what time, and in what location. This summary ensures that the child and the therapist are both clear on what will be tried, and children are more likely to remember plans that they have put into their own words. Sometimes spelling it out also reveals difficulties with the plan, as shown in the following example of a 10-year-old girl, Anita.

KM: Your new homework plan sounds really good and a lot less rushed than what you're doing now. Just so we're clear, can you spell out what you're going to do one last time?

ANITA: Sure. I am going to start my homework at 5:30 so that I have an hour before dinner, and then there will only be a little bit left after dinner to finish. That way, I'll have time to relax and chat with my friends in the evening.

KM: Sounds good. I'm glad you remembered your start time. Can you try that tomorrow night?

ANITA: Well, tomorrow night I have ballet; so, I'll have to eat dinner an hour early. Maybe I could try the next night.

KM: I'm not sure about that. Another possibility might be to make a different start time on ballet nights. Otherwise, you might not get to homework at all on those nights, and then it will pile up and you'll be rushing to finish it the following night.

ANITA: (*upset*) But then I don't get any downtime after school! It will just be school, then homework, then dinner, then ballet, and then my mom will make me go to bed.

KM: Is ballet important to you?

ANITA: Sure! I might even get a small part in "The Nutcracker" at Christmas this year. That would be amazing!

KM: Then, maybe it's worth giving up the downtime for ballet sometimes. What do you think?

ANITA: (*grumbling*) OK. I'll start homework at 4:00 on ballet nights. Why can't the school day be shorter?

KM: It just can't. Sorry. But you've done a really nice job planning your evenings. Maybe you can fit in some downtime on the weekends. In the meantime, give this plan a try, and tell me next time how the homework battle is going.

Notice that when I attach Anita's plan to a specific time (tomorrow night) she becomes aware of an obstacle that might prevent its implementation (ballet lessons) that she had not previously considered. Many children make plans that seem feasible in theory but are difficult to implement in the context of other day-to-day activities. Addressing obstacles to implementation is an important part of preparing the child to try out a new solution.

DIFFICULTIES AND CONTINGENCY PLANS

Sometimes difficulties with implementation arise unexpectedly, as in the example above, but often such difficulties can be anticipated. If you anticipate some problems with the child's plan, it is tempting to say, "That won't work because ... " and indicate the difficulties you expect. This is not very helpful, however, because it denies the child the opportunity to think about potential difficulties (and thus learn how to anticipate them), and it may sound discouraging to the child. Instead, it is usually more helpful to see if the child can anticipate the difficulties in response to a few leading questions. These may include:

- "What might stop you from doing that?"
- "What could get in the way of that plan?"
- "What would your friends say if you did that?"
- "What would your parents/family/teacher say if you did that?"
- "Is there anything else you need to do for that plan to work?"
- "Is there anyone else you need to talk to for that plan to work?"
- "Is there anything you could do if the plan didn't work?"

The last question alludes to another important aspect of preparing to try a new solution: having a contingency plan. This is especially important if the plan's chances of success are modest or if there is a small but acceptable risk associated with the plan. In the first case, it may be reassuring for the child to know that if the new solution cannot be implemented right away, all is not lost as there is a backup plan. In the second case, it may be reassuring to the child's parents to know that the therapist has put some thought into minimizing the risks associated with the child's plan.

For example, suppose a child decides to take a skiing lesson but has never tried the sport before and is worried about falling and being stuck halfway down the hill with skis twisted at odd angles, unable to get up. For a novice skier, the chances of this occurring are fairly high. A good contingency plan would be to talk to the instructor ahead of time to ensure the child will be helped up promptly, should this predicament arise. The child may be reassured that help is available "just in case" and therefore be more likely to take the lesson.

An example of a situation involving a small but acceptable risk is that of a 12- or 13-year-old child learning to let himself into the house after being dropped off by the school bus before his parents are home from work. Managing this situation can represent a nice step toward independence, but it also requires a contingency plan. For example, the child could forget or lose his house key. Anticipating this potential problem, his parents could leave a spare key with a trusted neighbor. They could also start the plan at a time of year when the weather is not too cold, so the child would be safe spending an hour or two outdoors if needed. Other families might have the child call a parent's cell phone upon arrival at the house to confirm his or her safe arrival. Whatever contingency plan is chosen, its goal would be to promote the child's independent coping at the end of the school day while minimizing risks. When they are reassured that they have planned for the worst, many families are able to hope for the best and allow their older children and adolescents to gradually act with greater autonomy.

PARENTAL SUPPORT

Some new solutions require the support of parents or other adults in order to be implemented successfully. This is more likely to be true if the child is young, debilitated by serious psychological problems (e.g., a significant mood disorder), or has demonstrated developmental delays that necessitate extra support. Support can include emotional support such as encouraging words, concrete assistance with the new solution (e.g., asking a teacher to monitor the child's progress in approaching other children in the playground at recess), or scaffolding.

Scaffolding occurs when adults implement part of the solution, allowing children to do only those parts that they are likely to be able to do successfully on their own. Then, gradually, children are permitted to implement more and more of the solution until they can implement the whole solution independently. When learning to cook, for example, we often allow children to help by having them read the recipes aloud, add the various ingredients we provide, and then stir them together. Once the children have mastered these basic tasks, we may also permit them to prepare some ingredients or to turn on the stove to the required temperature. Eventually, when they demonstrate proficiency at most of these tasks, we may allow them to do tasks that are more risky or challenging, such as chopping up vegetables or folding in beaten egg whites. Then, we may allow them to cook an entire meal without help, but with adult supervision. Then, and only then, will we allow them to cook meals completely independently.

Solutions that require adult support often make adults anxious. For example, the first time a child goes to overnight camp, the parent may have to do most of the packing, provide a list of emergency contact information for the camp in case there are unexpected problems, and speak to one or more counselors ahead of time regarding any special needs or difficulties the child may have that could affect the camp experience (e.g., bedwetting or food allergies). Within a few hours of arriving at camp, however, the child is usually less anxious than the parent. Furthermore, by the end of the stay at camp, many of the supports provided initially may no longer be needed. Thus, allowing children to venture into situations that challenge them to behave more independently is often helpful, and it ccontributes importantly to maturation. As therapists and parents, our challenge is to provide support without communicating too many of our own worries to the child.

Sometimes things do go wrong when children try solutions that have previously required parental support. For example, when packing for the return trip from camp, the child may often leave his or her toothbrush, socks, and other small items behind. A child who is just learning to use public transportation to get to school may forget or lose her bus fare occasionally. This situation is particularly common in children who have organizational difficulties caused by learning problems or ADHD. In most cases, we can empathize with the child's loss, encourage him or her to make lists or use other organizational strategies, and continue trying to improve the new solution.

If something more valuable is lost, however (e.g., a monthly bus pass worth $80), it night be tempting to dismiss the new solution and go back to the old one (e.g., driving the child to school). Think carefully, though, if there is a way of implementing the new solution with just a little extra support rather than forgoing it entirely. Perhaps the child can sort through change every morning and count out her bus fare for the day. Then, she can take the bus without risking the financial consequences of losing a monthly pass. Some independence has been gained, and she is also getting some extra practice with handling money. Similarly, the disorganized camper can be provided with a packing checklist, thus reducing the chances of leaving important items behind.

POSITIVE REINFORCEMENT

When children plan to try out new solutions, encourage them to give themselves credit regardless of the outcome. "Give yourself a pat on the back for trying something new/different/difficult" is one way to phrase this encouragement. Some children will jokingly give themselves a literal "pat on the back" when you say this, but most will get the idea. Trying anything new is hard work, and we need to give ourselves credit for this type of work.

Some children are perfectionist and will assume that they can only give themselves credit when they are completely successful. Talk to them about the value of partial success and of just trying their best. Sometimes it is OK to finish third in a race rather than first; to get a gift for someone even if their reaction tells you it was not exactly what they wanted; or to improve your swimming skills by taking a course even if you don't pass the final exam on the first attempt. By making the attempt to try these things, we learn and we grow. Learning and growing makes us stronger, regardless of the outcome. We can use that strength to persevere and make further, more successful, attempts or to try something different that we have a better chance of achieving. Either way, the effort is not wasted.

As therapists, we can also encourage any attempt to try a new solution. Sometimes success is its own reward, and anyway children are generally motivated by the intrinsic pleasure of achieving something new. This does not always happen, however; so, it is worth acknowledging the child's efforts with some praise. We can praise children's efforts in a meaningful way. Meaningful praise is sincere and *specific*. For example, "Confronting your math teacher about how you need her to explain things more slowly took courage. Not every student would dare to do that!" is more meaningful praise than "It's good you talked to your math teacher."

We can also provide points, stickers, or small prizes when children complete the "homework" of trying something new between sessions. Some children like a "point bank" or "prize bank" where they can see these items accumulate. Others prefer to enjoy them right away. Adolescents may prefer other types of rewards (e.g., a chance to talk about the attempt or about a topic of their choice, some time playing a game with you, a movie pass for several attempts). Time-based rewards (e.g., game time, talk time, or computer time) can be used with children of all ages. They are inexpensive and often valued as much or more than material rewards.

Children or adolescents sometimes claim that rewards don't matter to them. For these youngsters, however, meaningful praise is still perceived as rewarding. They may also be afraid that being thankful for a reward will result in the therapist's expecting them to do further work. If you suspect this issue applies, clarify the situation for the child or teen: "This is supposed to make *your life better*—whether or not it makes me happy." Then, see if the child or teen can find something intrinsically rewarding about the new solution. Changes that children make for their own benefit are more likely to last than those made to please their therapists.

Parents can also reinforce children's new solutions. This practice is particularly important when working with young children but can be helpful to some degree with children and adolescents of all ages. Some parents question this practice, wondering if they are bribing children to change. For these parents, I usually explain that a bribe is something offered in advance to induce someone to perform an illegal activity. A reward, on the other hand, is provided *after* a legitimate job is done well. A reward is much more similar to a paycheck at the end of the week than to a bribe.

Review the different types of rewards with parents: intrinsic rewards, meaningful praise, time-based rewards, and small material rewards (note: large material rewards are problematic because they are difficult to repeat, and most new behaviors must be repeated several times to become well established). Don't forget to discuss the value of rewarding partial success. We have all heard the old story of the child who came home with a 98% grade on the test and the parent who asked, "What happened to the other 2%?" Few comments are more discouraging.

Rely on parental wisdom and experience in finding out what a particular child considers most motivating or most rewarding. Parents have spent years with their children before they ever came to see a therapist; so, they usually have a good understanding of what "works" or "doesn't work" in trying to motivate their child. They know which hobbies their child pursues that could be supported with small rewards (e.g., stamps or coins for children who collect them, sports-focused or anime-based cards for children who prefer these).

One of the most difficult tasks for parents is to ignore setbacks. Parents may be quite good at responding positively when they see their children implementing new solutions, but they become very frustrated when their children occasionally revert to old habits. For example, a child may remember to bring home assignments four out of five school days, but when he or she forgets on that fifth day, the parent may respond with "Oh no! Not this again! I thought we were past all that!" Paradoxically, this sort of negative emotional reaction actually increases the chances of the next assignment's being forgotten as well. The child becomes upset, which can affect his or her ability to think clearly and focus on remembering assignments. Also, whether the child is aware of it or not, the extra parental attention derived from all that emotional interaction is a type of reinforcement for bad behavior; and reinforced behavior tends to be repeated.

How should the parent respond? Neutral is probably best. Some people cannot help but frown at a negative outcome, and that is probably OK, too. Encourage minimal talking and certainly no arguing or lecturing, as arguing and lecturing provide attention (i.e., a form of reward) for bad behavior (see above). "Oh, well, let's try again tomorrow—you're getting there" is probably the best response. This type of statement is mildly encouraging, reflecting the four good days so far. Nothing else, whether positive or negative, needs to be said.

WHEN NOTHING HAPPENS

Sometimes, despite ample preparation, new solutions are not implemented. If the child is reasonably cooperative, implementation within therapy sessions can be ensured, but implementation between sessions is a different story. Children often perceive trying a new solution in their daily lives as a type of homework, and (as any experienced teacher will attest) there are many, many excuses for not doing homework.

Trying to avoid or delay a new or challenging task is human nature, to some degree. Children or parents can forget to try a new solution, especially if they are distracted by other activities or events. There may be ambivalence about trying the new solution that has not been acknowledged to the therapist. Sometimes there is an obstacle to implementing a new solution that was not anticipated ahead of time. Trying to implement several new solutions at once can also be problematic, as most people can learn to do only one new thing at a time. Explore these possibilities when a child or parent sheepishly admits to not implementing the new solution they had agreed to put into practice at the end of the preceding session.

Specific emotional or behavioral problems can also interfere with children's and families' implementation of new solutions. Children who are inattentive are prone to forgetting tasks and losing items needed to complete tasks. Asking an inattentive child to use a day planner to help remember and organize school homework, for example, is often a good idea. However, day planners work only if children remember to bring them home each afternoon and bring them to school each morning. If they are lost or left behind, their utility is limited. If an inattentive child is asked to implement a new solution, adults may need to provide reminders or ensure that any items needed are available even if the child leaves them behind.

Depressed children and adolescents can also struggle to implement new solutions. Depression can interfere by reducing the child's energy level or result in distorted thinking that emphasizes personal helplessness. The latter problem, commonly termed "learned helplessness" (Nolen-Hoeksema, Girgus, & Seligman, 1986), occurs when someone assumes that he or she cannot influence the outcome of a situation before even trying to do so. It can occur either as a result of depressed thinking or repeated disappointment when trying to influence an outcome. Children with learning disabilities, for example, are often reluctant to attempt new academic tasks because they assume they cannot accomplish them. In this case, it is helpful to break a task into small chunks and have the child do each chunk with adult support and positive reinforcement for even the most minimal effort or participation. A patient but persistent approach is needed to encourage the child's gradually increasing efforts and thereby overcome his or her assumption of helplessness.

Anxious children are prone to avoiding anything they fear, and some fear almost all new situations or new challenges. They will not always acknowledge their fear, however, so the problem cannot always be anticipated. For example, a socially anxious boy who is working on overcoming his isolation may claim that he didn't go to a party because "that would be boring" or "I don't hang out with those guys." It is worth gently challenging these statements or at least asking what would have happened if he had gone to the party. The latter approach would result in some imagined exposure to the party (which is sometimes a helpful first step prior to actually attending) and might reveal what aspects of this situation are frightening the boy. Once the fear is acknowledged, the child and therapist can then problem-solve how it could best be addressed.

Anxious children may also avoid implementing new solutions owing to perfectionist tendencies. They may expect themselves to perform a new behavior perfectly on the first try. If they doubt their ability to do so, they may avoid trying the behavior in order to avoid failing to meet their own (unrealistic) standards. If you suspect that this perfectionist proclivity is to blame, talk about how it is normal to make some mistakes the first time you try something and how several tries are usually needed to accomplish a new task with complete success. If the child is really stuck, I sometimes resort to the old axiom "Doing something is always better than doing nothing" and treat the implementation of a new solution as an experiment. Even if the experiment fails, something is learned from it, and learning is a good thing. Thus, the child cannot lose by making an attempt.

Children with oppositional tendencies sometimes fail to implement new solutions if they feel that they have been pushed or coerced into trying them. Paradoxically, attempts to encourage these children sometimes backfire. For example, a well-meaning parent may say, "Suzy, it would be wonderful if you could get dressed on time every morning. We wouldn't have to argue or end up being late for school. Wouldn't that be nice?" If Suzy has oppositional tendencies, she might respond, "Nice for you, maybe, but what do I get out of it?" Rather than trying to either placate the child or challenge his or her oppositionality, it is often helpful to reframe the solution in a way that is consistent with the child's goals. If Suzy's goal is to get an extra 10 minutes of sleep, then showing her mother she can dress quickly may be helpful in that it will eventually result in a later wake-up time. The therapist's greatest challenge in working with these children is to get them to see the new solution as their own rather than as something being imposed by adults.

Sometimes we assume that the child's difficulties are preventing implementation of a new solution when in fact family factors are more to blame. Similar to their children, parents may forget, be ambivalent about the solution, encounter obstacles, or struggle with their own emotional difficulties. Explore these possibilities if the child appears to have tried to follow up but has encountered a lack of parental support.

Furthermore, parents may not realize that helping the child implement the new solution needs to be at the top of the family's priority list for at least the first few weeks or else it is unlikely to happen. Families' lives are busy, and parents often have myriad work, family, and social responsibilities. If the need to focus on the child's new solution is not written in bold letters and pasted on the refrigerator, it is often forgotten. Suggest such concrete visual reminders to families who struggle to support their children's progress. If the family cannot prioritize the child's solution because of more significant stresses (e.g., a serious illness in the family, an impending divorce, extreme poverty), defer the process until these critical family problems have been resolved.

Parents' volatile emotions can also prevent implementation of new solutions in some children. Anxious parents often worry that their children cannot manage a new solution or might be harmed in attempting it. For example, I have seen a number of teens who wanted to take public transit to their after-school activities but were only allowed to do so if they agreed to be accompanied by a parent, at least initially. Depressed parents may lack the energy to participate in their children's new solutions or (in some cases) may place a high value on having the child stay at home, thus interfering with children's best attempts to develop age-appropriate independence. They may also have difficulty encouraging their children or expressing confidence in their abilities, resulting in self-doubt in these children. Obviously, parents who struggle with inattention or disorganization may also have difficulty supporting their children's new solutions for these reasons.

LET'S TRY AGAIN

Whatever the reason for the lack of implementation of a new solution, avoid becoming angry with the child or the parents. It is natural to be frustrated when people confess that they did not work on their problem between sessions, especially if the therapist has carefully helped them prepare to implement the new solution (e.g., by using a checklist such as the one in Figure 6.1). However, becoming angry is rarely helpful and reduces the chances of learning why the solution was not implemented. Sensitive children or parents may even discontinue therapy if the therapist becomes angry.

Instead, express curiosity about what happened. Acknowledge the fact that it is unfortunate that nothing was done between sessions, since attempting the new solution would have been informative regardless of the outcome. Then explore the likely reasons for the lack of progress, listen empathetically to the person's response or suggested reasons, and only move on when you are certain that the reasons are clear. Sometimes, the reason offered is not something you would have expected, as the example of a 14-year-old girl, Mary, illustrates below.

> KM: I'm glad you decided last time to work on getting into better physical condition. I know you're hoping to reduce the teasing

about your weight, but it's a healthy thing to do regardless of what the other kids say about your appearance. Did you join a sport at school, as we discussed?

MARY: (*looking down*) No. I didn't get around to it.

KM: That's too bad. It would have been nice to have something to discuss and learn from. Did you forget?

MARY: (*nervously*) No, I tried. I even signed up for volleyball.

KM: What happened after you signed up?

MARY: I went to the first practice.

KM: Wow! That's great! How did it go?

MARY: (*blushing*) Not so good. I'm not going to go back.

KM: Did someone say something mean or make fun of you?

MARY: No. It's just not a good idea.

KM: What makes it a bad idea?

MARY: (*starting to cry*) It just is, that's all!

KM: (*offering a tissue*) I'm sorry it's so upsetting to talk about this. I understand if you don't want to go into detail, but can you give me a hint what the problem was? It might help to know so that we can avoid it in the future if we try something else. Is there anything you can share?

MARY: (*after a moment, taking a deep breath*) When I jumped, I had an accident with my top. I never want to show my face in that gym again.

KM: When you say "accident" you mean a problem with your bra. Is that right? (*Mary nods.*) No wonder you don't want to go back! You must have felt awful, and I'll bet your friends felt badly for you too.

MARY: Well, at least they didn't laugh.

KM: That's good. Maybe it's happened to one or two of them as well. I know it may feel like you're the only one this has happened to, but it's actually a common problem in girls your age. I think there are even sports bras you can get to reduce the chances of this happening.

MARY: My mother says we're only allowed to get new clothes at the start of the school year, and that was last month.

KM: I think she might make an exception for something like this. Would you like to talk to her together?

MARY: Yeah. That would be good.

Mary's mother understood her dilemma, purchased the sports bra, and encouraged her to try a different sport to avoid bad memories of the event. Mary agreed and joined in playing basketball, which she enjoyed. The example illustrates that we can't always assume that we know why our clients don't implement the solutions they agree to. By refraining from judgment before we have all the facts, we often allow them to feel safe enough to disclose what interfered with their plan. As in Mary's case, the obstacle may be relatively easy to address once it is clear what happened.

ANTICIPATING DIFFICULTIES WITH IMPLEMENTATION

Before moving on to the next chapter, it may be useful to practice anticipating possible difficulties that may arise when clients try to implement their new solutions. Therefore, I have reiterated below several examples from previous chapters. Using the information in this chapter, including Figure 6.1, try to anticipate possible problems with implementation in each case, and think about how you would address these. Ask yourself: "What could go wrong with this plan?", "What could I discuss with the client to improve the chances of success?", and "Is there anything I need to discuss with someone other than the client to improve the chances of success?"

1. Mark (the high school student from Chapter 1) decides to talk to his father about applying to an out-of-state college he prefers instead of applying to his father's preferred college.
2. Jason (the school-age boy from Chapter 2) finds that computer games distract him from doing his project. He decides to do the parts of his project that do not require a computer first and then move on to the computer-based parts.
3. Carrie (the school-age girl from Chapter 2) decides to talk to Kathy (whom she saw whispering with another girl) about whether or not they are still friends.
4. Jennifer (the teenager from Chapter 2) decides to reassure her parents about her wish to go out with friends by agreeing to take

along a cell phone and call if needed; agreeing to be back home by curfew; telling her parents where she's going and who will be driving; taking along money for a cab if needed; and allowing her parents to meet her friends.

5. Jeff (the 12-year-old boy from Chapter 3) "doesn't do any homework unless constantly reminded," according to his mother. Jeff agrees to do a predetermined amount of homework and then show it to his mother, and his mother agrees not to nag him.

6. Suzy (the 8-year-old girl from Chapter 3) relies excessively on her mother's help to start the school day, much to the principal's consternation. To foster Suzy's independence, the principal agrees to have a staff member meet Suzy at the door, and Suzy's mother agrees to spend less time dropping Suzy off.

Chapter 7

Step 5: Following Up and Evaluating Outcomes

The final step in the problem-solving process, following up and evaluating the outcome, draws on all the previous steps and sets the stage for the client and therapist's further work together. As they learn from the outcome, the client and therapist become aware of what else is needed: nothing more, more implementation of the same solution, "fine-tuning" of the solution to increase its effectiveness, or trying something else. Each possibility is described in this chapter and is related to its corresponding outcome(s) in a table provided later. Before looking at these possibilities, however, it is important to understand a bit more about the nature of evaluation.

ENSURING THAT EVALUATION HAPPENS

It is important to schedule a specific follow-up time whenever a new solution is tried. If problem solving is occurring as part of a weekly therapy, this is relatively easy. Simply remind the client that you will discuss the outcome of the new solution you've agreed upon at the next session. If appointments are less regular, set a specific time for follow-up, and make sure that it is feasible for the client.

Remember that the task of implementing the new solution and evaluating it is competing with many other tasks and events in the client's life and in the life of the family. In younger children, remind the parents as well as the children of the follow-up time, and make sure it is feasible for both. In adolescents, agreement with the young person may be sufficient, but anticipate competing demands. For example, high school examinations, field trips, and other events that are out of the ordinary may interfere with implementing a new solution, with follow-up, or with both.

ENSURING THE ACCURACY OF EVALUATION

To ensure an accurate evaluation of the new solution, ask about it in an open-ended way. Rather than asking "Did it work?" or "Did it not work?" (i.e., closed questions), ask "*How* did it work out?" or "What happened when you tried it?"(i.e., open-ended questions). If the response is vague, refer back to the baseline you recorded earlier in Chapter 3 (see pp. 39–40).

To review, changes from the baseline are any small signs of improvement in the situation you are addressing. These can include the child's getting through the stressful situation with less disruptive or less emotional behavior, acting more quickly, acting more slowly but more competently, or managing the situation more effectively or with greater confidence. If the child rated the initial level of difficulty of the situation or the level of distress it caused, ask him to redo the rating now, using a scale from 1 (easy) to 10 (very difficult or distressing).

It is important to elicit a detailed response so that you and the client can learn from the result, whatever it may be. This type of learning will facilitate decisions about what to do next (see below). For example, if an 8-year-old girl who is impulsive and is working on doing her homework slowly but accurately reports that "my teacher says I'm doing better," try to get a description of how she has done her homework in the past few days, including the time spent, the number of mistakes made, how easy or difficult it was for her to stay on task, and her level of comfort or discomfort with slowing down. If parents supervise her homework (as many do with children of this age), elicit their observations as well. In this case, we are not discounting the teacher's opinion. Rather, we are taking it as one piece of evidence that the girl is making progress but looking at other evidence as well. Thus, it is possible that the girl is doing better because she found the work assigned that particular week easy, because her parents decided to check her homework before it was handed in, or because she was doing it slowly and more carefully. Only the last possibility relates directly to her problem-solving efforts.

Detailed descriptions also make it easier to detect small signs of progress when the problem is not entirely solved, avoiding discouragement in children and parents. For example, a parent may say, "Nothing's changed. He's still anxious at bedtime." In this case, I might go back to a baseline description of the problem and ask, "Is it still taking about 2 hours to settle him at night?" or "Do you still have to physically wrestle with him to get him into his own bed?" If the child's period of distress is getting slightly shorter or if he is becoming a little bit more compliant at bedtime, these changes would suggest that his anxiety is starting to decrease. Detecting that small improvement is important if the child and family are to remain hopeful and persevere in working on the problem.

These changes may also suggest that the child is making an effort to improve his bedtime behavior or that the parents are making an effort to use a consistent bedtime routine. It is important for the therapist to positively reinforce these efforts in order to keep the child and family engaged in therapy and motivated to continue working on the problem. Conversely, if there really is no improvement despite everyone's best efforts, acknowledging this fact and responding empathetically can maintain the therapeutic alliance and still enable one to explore other solutions.

EVALUATION BIASES

The discussion above already suggests one possible bias when evaluating results: the "all-or-nothing" bias. Without a detailed evaluation, some people are prone to thinking about outcomes in only two categories: success or failure. As very few solutions work perfectly the first time you try them, these people often conclude that their efforts have resulted in failure even when they are starting to make progress. Not surprisingly, the "all-or-nothing" bias is common in people of all ages who are prone to depression. It can also occur in young or cognitively immature children, however, because it is simpler to think about two categories (i.e., success or failure) than about various degrees of improvement.

Another common bias in people prone to depression is one concerning attributions. People prone to depression tend to attribute success to circumstances or to "good luck" and failure to their own shortcomings. Thus, they have a difficult time giving themselves credit when they succeed and often blame themselves for perceived failures. People who are anxious may also have difficulty recognizing their own contributions to successful outcomes, usually because they underestimate their own capabilities.

Anxious people also sometimes confuse feelings and results, assuming that if they don't feel entirely confident in a situation then they have not handled the situation very well. There are many other thought biases or "cognitive distortions" that can occur, particularly in people with anxious or depressive tendencies (reviewed in Burns, 1999), but the three described above are most relevant to evaluating results. Below are some tips for addressing each of these biases:

THE ALL-OR-NOTHING BIAS

- Inquire about degrees of progress. For example, ask, "Was it even a little bit better/easier/less upsetting than last time?" or "Think back to how this situation was for you at the very beginning. If you compare what happened this week to how it was then, is there any difference (even a small one)?"
- Look at the baseline, and see if you can detect any sign of progress that the child or parents may have missed.
- Praise every effort, and reframe it as a sign of progress (i.e., you are always further ahead doing something than doing nothing). Do this even if efforts are less frequent than planned (e.g., one attempt a week vs. daily practice) or if the child has only done part of what was agreed upon.
- Normalize partial success, and encourage self-reward even if the result is not perfect. For example, say, "Sometimes even if you do a good job, things don't work out exactly as planned. Sometimes, you do OK but you might think you could have done a better job. Nobody's perfect, so give yourself a pat on the back for a really good try. That way, you won't give up and you can try again tomorrow!"
- The saying "practice makes perfect" is sometimes helpful. Remind the child that most people are not all-star athletes the first time they try a sport. Just like trying a new sport, trying a new solution takes practice. It may not work out perfectly the first time, but by practicing it the child can succeed in the long run.

THE ATTRIBUTIONAL BIAS

- Don't accept "It was just good luck" or "It was just an easy test" if the child succeeds. "You must have done something to get that result. What was it?" is a proper therapeutic response. Children need to learn to attribute success to their own efforts in order to persevere.

- When the result is disappointing, suggest that there are usually many reasons why things go wrong, and explore these. For example, say, "I know your hard work didn't seem to pay off this time, but what other reasons might there be for that result?"
- Don't accept "It's all my fault" if the child does not succeed. This sort of unqualified self-criticism is not helpful and can result in discouragement and despair. First, explore other reasons for the result. Then ask, "What could you have done differently?" This question refocuses the child on specific actions rather than personal shortcomings.

DISTINGUISHING FEELINGS AND RESULTS

- Remind the child that most people do better before they feel better; that is, feelings eventually get better as you become more competent at doing something.
- Praise the child's courage for trying to do something new despite being nervous or uncomfortable. It may also help to define courage: being courageous does not mean being fearless but rather doing what is important despite one's fears.
- If you have an objective measure of the results (e.g., a change from the baseline), use this measure as evidence that the child did well despite his or her uncomfortable feelings.
- If others have observed the child's new behavior, ask them to provide their observations. Children are sometimes surprised at how competent they appear to others even when they are feeling anxious.

POSSIBLE OUTCOMES AND NEXT STEPS

Once you have done an accurate, unbiased evaluation of the outcome, the next question is what to do with this information. The answer differs depending on what has been found. In Table 7.1, eight possible outcomes are listed along with a synopsis of corresponding therapeutic responses and next steps. Each will now be described and illustrated by referring back to some of the examples from the end of Chapter 6.

When No Attempt Has Been Made

From the therapist's point of view, the most potentially frustrating outcome is one where the client makes no attempt to implement the new

TABLE 7.1. Evaluating Outcomes

Client report back	Therapist response	Evaluation	Next step
No attempt	What happened?	Could not do it.	Problem-solve the obstacle.
No attempt	What happened?	Would not do it.	Address the client's motivation.
Attempt	Praise effort.	Problem solved.	What was learned?
Attempt	Praise effort.	Good progress.	What was learned? Keep working on it.
Attempt	Praise effort.	Some progress.	What was learned? Fine-tune and keep working on it.
Attempt	Praise effort.	Minimal progress.	What was learned? Fine-tune and keep working on it. *Or* Reevaluate the alternatives and consider trying a different one.
Attempt	Praise effort.	No progress.	What was learned? Reevaluate the alternatives and consider trying a different one.
Several cycles of attempts, fine-tuning, different alternatives, etc.	Praise perseverance.	No progress.	What was learned? Is this problem beyond the client's control? Consider accepting and making the best of the situation.

solution. Try to remain calm if this occurs, and review the section in Chapter 6 titled "When Nothing Happens" to see if you can understand the reasons for this outcome. Pay particular attention to any aspects of the child's emotional or behavioral problems that may be preventing successful implementation and to any ambivalence in the family about the new solution proposed. Try to avoid interpreting this outcome as a personal failure. As therapists, we are not responsible for making sure our client's problems are solved but rather for guiding their problem-solving efforts in as helpful a manner as possible.

A curious, nonjudgmental attitude is often helpful in addressing lack of implementation with the child and family. Ask, "What happened?", "What stopped you from doing it?", or "What made it difficult to try it this week?" The answers should help clarify whether there was a realistic obstacle to implementation (i.e., it couldn't be done), a lack of motivation to work on the new solution (i.e., the client/family wouldn't do it), or both.

Obstacles can come in several forms. Sometimes there is a lack of opportunity to try a new behavior. For example, a child may have rehearsed a new approach to deal with a child who is teasing him on the school bus, but if his tormentor is sick that week there is no opportunity to try the new approach. Sometimes there is an unexpected roadblock preventing implementation. For example, a family may decide to practice having their child walk home and let herself into the house after school independently, but the school may not allow her to leave the property unaccompanied without a permission form from the parents. Sometimes the child needs additional support from parents, school personnel, peers, or other people in order to try a new solution. These supports may need to be organized before trying the new solution again.

Sometimes children and families describe obstacles that are really reflective of a lack of motivation. For example, "We forgot to do it" or "We had a really busy week" typically indicate an inability to prioritize the child's problem-solving efforts rather than true obstacles. People tend to feel embarrassed about saying "We don't want to do it" or "We didn't feel like doing it," and so faulty memory and a busy lifestyle are blamed.

In this case, it may not be helpful to create memory aids or schedules or other tools to overcome the stated "obstacles." Instead, assume that there is a motivational issue and proceed accordingly. Try to empathize with the client's uncertainty about trying something new. Most people are ambivalent about change. Then refer back to some of the questions about motivation listed in Chapters 2 and 6.

Experts in motivation have described the goal of such questions as "creating a discrepancy between present behavior and important personal goals and values" (Miller & Rollnick, 2002). In other words, if the old way of doing things seems comfortable and the new solution does not relate to important personal goals or values, people are unlikely to change. Perhaps the child or parent does not see a great need to solve the problem at this time because the problem is not very distressing. Perhaps there is a need to further explore the value of trying a different approach. Either way, the therapist should not rush into another attempt to implement the new solution without making sure that the client (or client and parents, in the case of younger children) is eager to do so.

For example, suppose that Mark (the high school student from Chapter 1) has decided to talk to his father about applying to an out-of-state college he particularly likes instead of applying to his father's preferred college. He returns to his next session and shifts in his chair uneasily.

KM: (*after some small talk about the weather*) So, Mark, I'm curious to hear how it went when you talked to your father.

MARK: Uh, actually, I didn't get to talk to him. He was working the nightshift this week, so I didn't have a chance.

KM: How do you feel about that?

MARK: Well, I'm glad I didn't have to face him, but it's getting close to the deadline for applications, so I guess I'm worried too.

KM: So, you're safe for the moment but kind of stressed about what comes next.

MARK: Exactly!

KM: So, where do you go from here?

MARK: Do you think I should try talking to him again?

KM: Only if you're sure that's what you want to do. If you'd rather look at some of the other alternatives we discussed earlier, we could do that too.

MARK: We've been talking about this for weeks now! It's like a big cloud hanging over my head.

KM: You're getting tired of this issue, and that's hard, but it's still not resolved. What would help?

MARK: (*thinking for a moment*) If I wasn't such a chicken. My dad's gonna find out eventually, and he'll be more angry if I try going behind his back. I should be a man and face him.

KM: That's a tough choice. Are you OK with it?

MARK: It's the only choice. I'm talking to him tonight.

Therapists focused on problem solving usually like to help clients find solutions. When someone is ambivalent about a solution (as Mark is), however, advocating too strongly for that solution can backfire. Instead, try to ask some leading questions and to avoid directly telling the client what to do. You may have to bite your tongue to avoid making suggestions (I often do), but the end result is that the client feels more committed to whatever solution is pursued. For a more detailed description of how to do this, see Miller and Rollnick's (2002) classic book *Motivational Interviewing: Preparing People for Change*.

When the Problem Is Solved

Sometimes, children report that they have implemented a new solution and the problem is solved. If it happens, it is tempting to simply rejoice and send them on their way. However, this might result in the child's showing up with a very similar problem a few weeks or a few months later, seeking another solution. Instead, find out exactly what happened and how the child contributed to the positive outcome. This allows you to do two things: provide effective praise that is specific to the child's contribution and learn how the positive outcome can be maintained or repeated in similar situations.

For example, suppose that Carrie, a school-age girl, decides to talk to Kathy (whom she saw whispering with another girl) about whether or not they are still friends. She reports back the next week that the problem is solved and she has just returned from a wonderful sleepover with Kathy.

> KM: Wow! You went from suspecting Kathy of saying bad things about you, to being really good friends again. How did you do that?
>
> CARRIE: It wasn't all me. I asked Kathy what she was talking about, and she told me: she was asking what I might like for my birthday! I sure felt bad for thinking she was badmouthing me. She got me a really nice present, too. Then I gave her a big hug.
>
> KM: So, you had the courage to ask her for an explanation and then the good sense to stop suspecting her and welcome her back as a friend. Good job! What did you learn from this experience?
>
> CARRIE: To get the facts before I start to blame my friends for stuff.
>
> KM: Yup. Anything else?
>
> CARRIE: That I have some really good friends, like Kathy, and I should hang onto them.
>
> KM: Great. Those sound like some really good lessons. Do you want to share them with anyone?
>
> CARRIE: My mom, I guess. I know she was worried about me.

Carrie may or may not remember these lessons in her next encounter with peers, but she has clearly gained some confidence in her ability to solve problems related to her peer group. She is also willing to share her experience with her mother. This sharing may increase her mother's confidence in her daughter's problem-solving ability (allowing her to positively reinforce it) and allow Carrie's mother to remind her of this experience in the future if a similar situation arises.

When There Is Substantial Progress

Few problems are completely solved with the first attempt to address them. Most problems require repeated efforts; so, it is important to acknowledge and positively reinforce those efforts. When there is substantial progress, nothing more may be needed. On the other hand, sometimes a bit of "fine-tuning" can result in even greater progress on the next attempt; so, it is still important to find out exactly what happened. Then decide if the client should be encouraged to do "more of the same" or "more of something very similar" (i.e., minor modification of the strategy).

As mentioned before, effective praise is specific to the situation and the person's efforts to address it. Thus, comments like "That's impressive. Your idea worked better than expected" or "Wow! That strategy's a keeper" are more specific and therefore often more helpful than just "Good job" or "Nice result." Focusing on the strategy also leads naturally into talking about its repetition, encouraging the child to do more of the same until the problem is solved.

Encourage the child to self-evaluate as well. "Are you pleased with this result?" is sometimes a good question to ask. Self-evaluation reduces dependency on the therapist for this problem-solving step and often helps children discover the intrinsic satisfaction of a job well done. This satisfaction can improve future motivation.

Self-evaluation is particularly important for adolescents, who may perceive some evaluative comments by the therapist as patronizing or condescending. Imagine the look on a 15-year-old's face when an adult says to him, "Good boy!" Most adolescents would cringe at this type of remark. Self-evaluative questions are much more respectful of their autonomy.

If multiple repetitions of the same solution will be needed or if the task makes the child somewhat uncomfortable, consider tracking the child's efforts and/or attaching tangible rewards to these efforts. Remembering to bring home one's homework is an example of something needing multiple repetitions; desensitizing an anxious child to a particular phobia is an example of a somewhat uncomfortable task. Nobody enjoys doing tedious or uncomfortable tasks, but sometimes they are necessary.

Rewarding effort with a star or sticker on a chart is often help-ful for younger children. The chart provides a visual reminder of prog-ress, which is encouraging, and the stars and stickers improve the chil-dren's motivation. It is important to minimize emphasis on setbacks, as emphasis on these can be discouraging or result in children arguing about whether or not a setback occurred. Therefore, lack of progress is indicated by not affixing a star or sticker and minimizing discussion, not by using an "X" or other negative mark on the chart.

Sometimes a larger reward is offered every 5 or 10 stickers, if this has been agreed upon in advance. Children have a very short time per-spective, so having to wait for more than 10 stickers usually makes the reward seem impossibly far away. Rewards should not be considered "bribes" (a common concern among parents), as they are provided only *after* children demonstrate effort, not before.

Stars and stickers are usually not considered meaningful by ado-lescents, but other forms of rewards can be used in this age group. An extra privilege (for example, extra computer time or being allowed to stay out an extra hour), a favorite activity, or some money toward an item of the adolescent's choosing are sometimes appropriate rewards. Reward systems for anxious children and youth are described in more detail in my parenting book about this population (Manassis, 2007). Not all children and teens need rewards to implement their solutions, however; so, use them only when praise and intrinsic motivation are not sufficiently motivating.

Before moving on, let's look at an example of responding to a child who is making substantial progress but needs to implement his solution repeatedly, with only minor modifications. Recall Jason (the school-age boy cited Chapter 2), who found that computer games distracted him from doing his project. He decided to do the parts of his project that do not require a computer first and then move on to the computer-based parts.

> KM: Last week, we talked about that project you were struggling with. Do you remember what you were going to try to do with that?
>
> JASON: Yup. I was going to do everything that I didn't need a com-puter for first.
>
> KM: You remembered! Is that what you actually did?
>
> JASON: Yup. I organized it and wrote it all out by hand, turned on the computer, and then... it still took 3 more hours to finish.

KM: Sounds like you followed your strategy really well and finished the project. Good work! [I offer specific praise.] Were you pleased with the result or still concerned about how long that last step took? [I encourage self-evaluation and learning some more from this experience.]

JASON: I got off-track at the end: I took 3 hours to type three pages and didn't get to sleep 'til after midnight. But, you see, as soon as I turned on the computer, I saw the "You've got mail" sign, and I had to check my messages, and then so much was happening with my friend Joe that I started responding ...

KM: ... and then you got distracted from your project.

JASON: Yup. Foiled again by the computer! [He shows a bit of all-or-nothing thinking here.]

KM: Still, you stayed on track for most of the project. [I try to correct the all-or-nothing bias.] What could you do differently next time? [I encourage fine-tuning.]

JASON: I guess I could turn off that automatic "You've got mail" function. That way, I could finish and *then* check my mail.

KM: Sounds like a plan. One or two more projects, and this way of working will come automatically. Great start! [I offer positive reinforcement and encouragement to continue implementing his strategy with only a minor modification.]

Fine-Tuning

"Fine-tuning" is an approach used in situations where things are going well but could be going even better. Most people trying something new do not perform it perfectly the first time. Sometimes they need more practice. Sometimes they also need some coaching on how to do the new task more effectively. When a therapist provides such coaching to help a client implement a new solution more effectively, this practice is termed "fine-tuning."

Fine-tuning is particularly helpful in situations where there has been substantial progress (suggesting that the solution attempted has some merit) but the outcome is less than perfect. For example, we saw a need to "fine-tune" Jason's approach, above, as he got distracted by an automatic computer function. In this case, the modification needed was immediately obvious to the client (i.e., to turn off the mail notification function). In other cases, the modification needed may not be obvious to the client but be easily recognized by the therapist.

For example, recall Jennifer (from Chapter 2), a teen who decided to reassure her parents about her wish to go out with friends by doing the following: agreeing to take along a cell phone and call if needed, agreeing to be back by curfew, telling them where she's going and who would be driving, taking along money for a cab if needed, and allowing her parents to meet her friends. While Jennifer's intentions are admirable, the number of additional tasks she is hoping to do to reassure her parents may be impossible to remember without a checklist! Moreover, some of the tasks would require her parents' participation (namely, meeting her friends and obtaining money for the cab).

Simplifying a solution and getting others to assist with implementation are two common examples of "fine-tuning" strategies that can improve the chances of a solution's success. Some others include removing an obstacle to implementing the solution (e.g., the "You've got mail" computer function, mentioned above); spelling out the details of implementation more precisely (i.e., who is going to do what, at what time, and where); ensuring that the solution is implemented consistently by all people involved and at all times, increasing the frequency or duration of implementation (i.e., practice makes perfect); and addressing ambivalence about the solution in those around the client (for example, even the most motivated children sometimes abandon solutions their parents do not wholeheartedly support).

Even apparently simple solutions can require these types of "fine-tuning." For example, suppose that Terry, an 11-year-old boy who feels socially isolated at school, decides to try connecting with his peers by joining the school chess club. On the surface, this seems like a simple and feasible solution. However, upon closer examination, it becomes evident that the chess club practices regularly over the lunch hour (with no food allowed in the practice room) and tournaments occur at the end of the school day. Terry has problems with fine motor control; so, he requires more time than usual to eat his lunch. Thus, he can either eat his lunch and miss his practice or, alternatively, attend his practice and consume minimal amounts of food, potentially impacting his academic work in the afternoon. Furthermore, he takes a bus to and from school and requires a note from his parents whenever he intends to miss the bus. Thus, when there are tournaments, he must remember to ask his parents for a note for the bus, deliver that note to the office at school, and either ask a friend to get a ride home with him or make sure his parents can make alternate transportation arrangements. Forgetting to do any one of these things makes his attendance at tournaments impossible.

Terry's participation in the chess club will likely be erratic as a result of these logistical issues. If he is to benefit from this social connection, some "fine-tuning" may be needed. For example, it would be important for Terry's therapist to meet with his parents to make sure that they are in agreement with his participation in the club, can facilitate his transportation home from tournaments, and are willing to address (or allow the therapist to address) the school's procedures around lunchtime. Terry himself may have to write the dates for tournaments in his day planner as soon as they are available to make sure he remembers to obtain the required note for the bus.

When There Is Minimal or No Progress

When there has been an attempt to implement a new solution but progress is limited, the therapist faces a decision: either to work with the client to fine-tune the current solution in the hope of increasing its effectiveness or to encourage the client to try another solution. The choice requires some judgment, but a detailed description of what happened is always a good place to start. If the description suggests some way of either making the solution more effective (e.g., simplifying it, making it more precise, implementing it more consistently or more frequently) or of making the environment more conducive to its effectiveness (e.g., removing obstacles, getting others to help or at least not interfere with the solution), then it may be possible to fine-tune the solution and try again.

Modifying a solution is often preferable to trying something completely different, because it is usually less disruptive to the client's current routines and lifestyle and it avoids giving up on potentially successful solutions prematurely. Many therapists encounter families who say, "We've tried [or our child has tried] everything to solve this problem, and nothing has worked." A careful history usually reveals that a variety of solutions have been implemented, but often briefly, inconsistently, or in an environment where success would be unlikely.

Modifying a solution and trying again may not be advisable in those situations where a solution has had unexpected adverse results. For example, if a child has decided to assert his or her wishes about a particular situation and the other person responds with hostile, belittling comments, it may not be wise to encourage further assertiveness in that situation, as this may result in further exposure to verbal abuse or worse. In this case, a different approach to the situation is clearly needed.

Modifying a solution and trying again may also be inadvisable if the child is convinced that the solution cannot be helpful. He or she might say something like "I tried and it was impossible. I don't want to set myself up for another failure." While it is true that there may be some biased thinking contributing to such statements, the depth of the child's conviction suggests that it may be difficult to get him or her to try this particular solution again. A solution that is less challenging or that breaks the challenge into small steps may be worth considering in this case.

Regardless of the reasons for abandoning a solution, it is important to learn from it before moving on to the next one. Examining the unsuccessful attempt in detail and learning from it is helpful because it allows the child and therapist to avoid repeating any pitfalls or mistakes that occurred. This type of review also enables the therapist to reframe the unsuccessful attempt as a learning opportunity rather than a failure. Children are more likely to persevere if they realize that no effort is wasted, because all efforts can result in learning and therefore can improve the chances of future success.

Sometimes the reasons the attempt failed can even point the way to a different, more successful, solution. For example, if a child was unable to join a game with a group of peers in the schoolyard because of shyness about approaching them, perhaps bringing a game to school that others would find interesting might work better (as the other children would be approaching the shy child).

If the new solution is not obvious, go back to the alternatives generated in the second problem-solving step and reexamine these with the client to determine which one might be worth trying next. Look back at Figure 1.1 in Chapter 1. As the upward arrow indicates, in the event of an unsuccessful outcome, you resume with Step 2 and begin repeating the last several problem-solving steps with the client until a more successful solution is found.

For example, recall the case of Suzy (from Chapter 3), the 8-year-old girl who relied excessively on her mother's help to start the school day. The principal was quite frustrated with this behavior. To foster Suzy's independence, he agreed to have a staff member meet Suzy at the door, and Suzy's mother agreed to spend less time dropping Suzy off. During the first week, Suzy's mother went with the staff member and Suzy to the classroom and then sneaked out partway through the morning. Suzy was fine, but the staff member was annoyed and indicated that good-byes were to be said at the school door the following week.

That week, Suzy had daily tantrums at the school door, and her mother complained that the staff member was becoming verbally abusive toward her. After carefully examining exactly what was happening, it became clear that prolonged good-byes, regardless of the location, generally made Suzy's tantrums worse. This seemed to be the main reason for the lack of progress in this case. Unfortunately, Suzy's mother was not willing to consider a very brief good-bye from her daughter, as she feared her daughter would interpret this as being abandoned to the "cruel" school staff. Thus, fine-tuning the approach was unlikely to succeed.

Looking back at alternatives that had been generated early in the problem-solving process, there was one option that seemed to address this dilemma: having Suzy's father drop her off. The advantages of this option included that Suzy was generally less clingy with her father and that he tolerated brief good-byes from his daughter as long as there was a responsible adult present who could look after her. The main disadvantage was that he would have to change his work schedule to implement this solution. He was, however, willing to do so. Within a month of trying this option, Suzy was attending school with minimal distress and no longer needing the school staff member's support.

When Things Seem to Be "Stuck"

Sometimes even after several possible solutions have been attempted to address a problem, progress remains elusive. This dilemma is described in more detail in the final chapter of this volume, but is also addressed briefly here. When there is lack of progress after repeated attempts, it worth praising client perseverance but also trying to ascertain the reasons for the impasse. Some helpful questions for therapists in this situation include:

- Is solving the problem beyond the client's physical or intellectual abilities (at least for the time being)?
- Is an unacknowledged problem with client motivation preventing resolution of the problem?
- Does the client have too little influence or control in this situation to solve the problem?
- Are there others who are (either deliberately or inadvertently) undermining the client's efforts?
- Are there undiagnosed psychological problems in the child, other family members, or the family system that are interfering with progress?

To illustrate the last point, recall the case of Jeff (from Chapter 3), the 12-year-old boy who "doesn't do any homework unless constantly reminded," according to his mother. Jeff agrees to do a predetermined amount of homework and then show it to his mother, and his mother agrees not to nag him. You see Jeff and his mother a few weeks later.

MOTHER: (*sarcastically*) Well, we're back again. More fun and games with homework.

KM: I'm glad you're continuing to work on it. Remind me how you were trying to address the issue this week.

JEFF: (*interrupting*) She was supposed to back off, but she didn't!

KM: And what were you supposed to do?

JEFF: Show her my work. But it's never enough for her! She keeps telling me to do more. And on days when I don't have any homework, she doesn't believe me.

MOTHER: That's because when I called the teacher he told me Jeff is still not finishing his assignments on time.

KM: You were checking up on him?

MOTHER: Of course! How else could I get at the truth? He never tells me. I can't let him throw his future away!

KM: We've tried several different ways of improving the homework situation now, but I think we're talking about more than homework here. The amount of negative stuff that comes up when we talk about it suggests it may just be one example of a bigger problem. Jeff, you seem really hurt that your mother doesn't trust you in this area.

JEFF: (*interrupting*) She doesn't trust me at all.

KM: You care about what she thinks of you, Jeff. And Mrs. A., you seem genuinely worried about how your son's life will turn out if you do not keep tabs on him. You obviously care about him a great deal. Unfortunately, even though you both care, all that hurt and worry is coming out as anger and arguments. Are there any times where you enjoy your time together?

MOTHER: Not any more. If I took the time to enjoy, his grades would go south.

KM: You miss how it used to be.

MOTHER: Yeah, and he's not even a teenager yet! I dread what's coming.

KM: Being a parent certainly isn't easy, and the tricky part is the strategies that work with younger children sometimes backfire as they get older. And it's not easy for kids either. You probably want to be more independent now than in the past, Jeff, but you also want to feel your mother trusts and believes in you. I think some family counseling to work on how you relate to each other and communicate may be helpful. Sometimes problems like homework completion solve themselves once people are communicating more effectively.

In this case, I pursue one option for seemingly insoluble problems: I recommend another form of intervention that (I believe) is more likely to facilitate progress than continued problem solving. Other options may become apparent in response to the questions for therapists at the beginning of this section. Occasionally problems are encountered that cannot be remedied, despite our best efforts. In this case, accepting that fact and helping the client adapt to the situation may be the most therapeutic approach. As human beings, we all have limited control over the events of our lives. In childhood and old age, the limits to our control are most obvious, but they exist at all ages. Living within those limits with grace is not easy, but it is sometimes the wisest solution.

Chapter 8

Combining Problem Solving with Other Interventions

Having reviewed the component steps of problem solving, I can now turn to the bigger picture: integrating and combining problem solving with other interventions that may be part of your client's treatment plan. There are several variations on this theme. For example, problem solving can be included as one of several techniques in psychotherapy. In fact, it is already a component of some manualized treatments. In other situations, therapy with a problem-solving focus may be combined with other elements of the treatment plan (e.g., combining it with another form of psychotherapy or with a pharmacological treatment). Each of these three possibilities—that is, (1) including problem solving in therapy, (2) combining problem solving with another form of therapy, or (3) combining problem solving with a pharmacological treatment—poses unique challenges, and therefore a thoughtful approach is required. Table 8.1 outlines some of these challenges, which will be illustrated in this chapter by using specific examples.

INCLUDING PROBLEM SOLVING IN THERAPY

Several evidence-based treatments already contain some problem-solving elements, although they vary in the degree to which these are

TABLE 8.1. Combining Problem Solving with Other Interventions

Approach	Considerations
Including problem solving in psychotherapy	• Don't "dilute" the other therapy; instead, add sessions that are focused on problem solving. • Remember to follow up and evaluate outcomes, even if problem solving is not the main focus of a particular session. • Write down successful solutions so that the client can refer back to these. • Use problem solving to address realistic challenges that arise during therapy. • Use problem solving to apply therapeutic insights outside the office. • Use problem solving to overcome therapy obstacles.
Combining problem solving with another psychotherapy	• Don't overburden the client with therapy appointments, as this may result in fatigue, resistance, and concerns about stigma. • Communicate regularly with the other therapist. • Make sure therapies do not work at cross-purposes. • Consider doing therapies in sequence rather than concurrently (e.g., addressing the most realistic problem first; addressing low motivation or skills deficits first).
Combining problem solving with psychotropic medication(s)	• Consider combining these in severely impaired children. • Consider a short trial of problem solving in families that want medication only as a last resort or where children are less severely impaired. • Medication makes some children more amenable to problem solving or increases the range of solutions they are willing to consider. • Problem solving may aid decisions about medication and improve medication adherence. • Successful problem solving sometimes decreases the need for medication and improves self-efficacy. • Explore the psychological meaning of medication versus psychotherapy for the child and family, providing education if needed. • Be alert for medication side effects that may affect problem solving. • Medication that eliminates all symptoms may reduce the motivation to engage in problem solving. • Consider stabilizing medication before starting problem solving, to avoid the client's attributing all changes to medication or to problem solving. • Communicate regularly with the prescribing physician and consider a case conference if stuck.

emphasized and practiced. The time spent on problem solving may be relatively brief, however, and some children can benefit from additional work on problem-solving techniques. If so, it is important to add sessions for this purpose rather than "diluting" other elements of the treatment.

For example, common manuals for cognitive-behavioral therapy (CBT) for anxious children and adolescents (e.g., Kendall's [2006] "Coping Cat" manual for young anxious children and Kendall, Choudhury, Hudson, & Webb's [2002] "C.A.T. Project" manual for anxious adolescents) routinely combine cognitive restructuring and problem-solving techniques. Children are taught a "FEAR plan" of four steps that focuses on identifying anxiety, identifying anxious thoughts, finding helpful thoughts and actions to cope with a given anxious situation, and evaluating the result. Finding helpful actions that are put into practice in anxious situations and then evaluated can be thought of as a problem-solving process. However, if children focus exclusively on finding helpful actions (e.g., distracting themselves when facing feared situations or using deep breathing to calm themselves) and do not also learn to find helpful thoughts (e.g., asking themselves "What's the worst that can happen?" or remembering past successes in similar situations), an important element of CBT (i.e., cognitive restructuring) is lost.

Sometimes additional time needs to be spent on problem solving to address a realistic challenge that arises in therapy. For example, a 16-year-old boy who had been diagnosed with generalized anxiety disorder was doing CBT and, by using cognitive restructuring, had learned to manage his worries about examinations and large assignments. Then, however, he developed infectious mononucleosis, an illness that caused him to miss over a month of school. Using his cognitive strategies, he was able to reassure himself that he would be able to catch up on the work he missed. Figuring out *how* to catch up, however, required some problem solving. He eventually decided to talk to each of his teachers about what he needed to do and to obtain revised deadlines for assignments as well as notes from his friends. He also arranged for tutoring in his worst subject (chemistry), where he felt hopelessly confused. His therapist wisely decided to spend three sessions on this realistic challenge before resuming his focus on cognitive restructuring.

When including problem solving in psychotherapy, the therapist should guard against neglecting important elements of problem solving owing to the need to attend to other aspects of therapy. For example, if problem solving is the main focus of only one or two sessions, it is easy for the therapist to forget to follow up and evaluate the results of new solutions that have been tried out by the child between sessions. Without such evaluation, the benefits of problem solving are limited. Writing down successful solutions so that these are available to the child in the future is another helpful strategy when time spent on problem solving in therapy is brief.

Some therapies include problem solving as a means of applying what has been learned in therapy outside of the office. Interpersonal therapy, for example, encourages problem solving to address interpersonal problems once these have been identified and explored with the therapist. Interpersonal therapy has been found to be particularly helpful with depressed adolescents (Mufson, 2009; Santor & Kusamakar, 2001). Common therapy themes include role conflict, role transition, interpersonal loss, and interpersonal deficits. Examples of each include an adolescent stressed by differences between parental expectations of behavior and those of peers (role conflict), an adolescent facing new expectations of independent behavior when starting high school (role transition), an adolescent whose first serious romantic relationship ends (interpersonal loss), and an adolescent on the autistic spectrum who feels awkward or inept when relating to peers (interpersonal deficit). The client's predominant theme is identified and explored with the therapist, but successfully addressing the problem outside the therapist's office usually requires some problem solving. Dialectical behavior therapy uses problem solving in a similar manner, but usually in more severely troubled adolescents (e.g., severe personality disturbance, eating disorders, substance abuse) (Paris, 2010).

Consider the example of Anne, a 14-year-old girl who saw an interpersonal therapist after being diagnosed with dysthymic disorder (a chronic but mild form of depression), which she attributed to feeling "used" by her peers. Anne was very shy but highly intelligent and academically successful. Because of her shyness, she had difficulty making friends but was often approached by her peers for assistance with homework assignments. Eager to make friends, she readily provided help, but once the work was done they did not interact with her further. Anne was becoming discouraged about ever making friends, began avoiding her peers, and described feeling bitter. Her therapist identified role conflict as a theme (i.e., wanting to be liked by her peers but also wanting to like and respect herself). After a few sessions exploring this theme, the therapist encouraged Anne to look at alternative behaviors in relation to her peers that might further her goal of making true friends who were not just looking for extra help with their school work. She considered saying "No" to all peer requests for help with schoolwork, saying "Yes" only to those peers who had spent time with her outside of school, and asking for payment from those who asked for help. She eventually decided on the second alternative. Initially, she was only interacting with two peers (the two who had spent time with her outside of school at least once), but eventually they introduced her to other academically successful students, and she developed a circle of friends who helped one another with schoolwork as well as spent time together socially.

Some therapies (e.g., those focused on psychodynamic issues or family dynamics) do not contain an explicit problem-solving component. However, problem solving can sometimes be included in these therapies to overcome therapeutic obstacles. To do so, the therapist may need to temporarily shift to a more directive therapeutic stance than is usual for these therapies.

Consider the example of John, a 6-year-old boy who was treated in play therapy for posttraumatic symptoms arising from a house fire in which his brother died and he was badly burned. John's symptoms appeared to be improving, but his parents noticed that he became increasingly anxious as the summer approached and he insisted on continuing to wear winter clothing. When they tried to change him into short-sleeved shirts, he would have temper tantrums. He could not (or would not) explain why he did not want to wear summer clothes. John's therapist guessed that he might be concerned about others' reactions to the burn scars on his arms. The therapist role-played with John what he could say to a friend who asked about his scars, using a problem-solving approach. Then, he encouraged John's parents to invite one of his friends to the house so that John could practice his solution in a comfortable environment. After this experience, John's fear of wearing summer clothes subsided, and he was able to successfully complete his course of play therapy.

COMBINING PROBLEM SOLVING
WITH OTHER PSYCHOTHERAPIES

Some practitioners use psychotherapy focused primarily on problem solving as a stand-alone treatment. If the client is ready to problem-solve (see Chapter 2) and the challenges the client faces are amenable to problem solving (see Chapters 1 and 2), this can be a very helpful approach. When combining this type of therapy with other psychotherapies, however, several issues need to be considered. These are summarized in Table 8.1.

First, it is important not to overburden the client and his or her family with therapy appointments. This is especially relevant when working with children, as therapy appointments often compete with the child's other after-school activities and preadolescent children usually need to be transported to appointments by their parents. For children who struggle at school, afterschool activities, may be an important source of self-esteem and contributor to the child's quality of life. By depriving them of such activities, frequent therapy appointments can sometimes inadvertently contribute to children's unhappiness. Children may also experience increased fatigue, resistance to participating in therapy, and worries about stigma when participating in multiple therapies concurrently. For example, a child may be able to explain one appointment a week to friends as a regular doctor's visit (as many children with chronic illnesses require these) but is likely to encounter suspicion and questions among friends if there are multiple appointments per week. In addition, parents' work life may be adversely affected by frequent therapy appointments, and quality family time may also be reduced.

Sometimes there is a role for combining child-focused problem solving with another therapy involving other family members. In families where parental conflict contributes to the child's difficulties, for example, concurrent marital therapy may be helpful. Similarly, in families where a parent suffers from a significant mental illness, it may be helpful to find a therapist who can treat that parent's illness in addition to providing therapy with a problem-solving focus to the child.

Usually when the child is involved in more than one concurrent therapy, there is also more than one therapist. This fact raises a second issue: the need for regular communication with the other therapist. Communication is needed to ensure that therapies do not work at cross-purposes, to avoid providing mixed messages to the child and family, to avoid scheduling conflicts, and to determine who will be responsible for the overall treatment plan. This last issue is particularly important when working with children, as school personnel and other professionals may need to be involved in the child's care. When multiple people outside the child's family are involved, identifying a case manager who is responsible for the overall treatment plan permits better coordination among professionals.

Potential Conflicts with Other Therapies

From the examples above, which described ways of including problem solving with other therapies, it may appear that problem solving is compatible with most other psychotherapies. In general this is true, but occasionally therapists may find themselves disagreeing or working at cross-purposes. Some psychodynamic therapists, for example, may consider problem solving superficial because it focuses on implementing practical solutions for problems rather than on discovering their root causes. Both approaches, however, may have a role to play in helping children and adolescents.

For example, I once treated a high school student who worried constantly about either falling behind in school or not meeting the expectations of her peers in one of the numerous extracurricular activities she engaged in. Using a problem-solving approach, she was able to set priorities and better organize her schedule, but a month later she seemed to have even more tasks on her plate and was once again overwhelmed. It eventually became clear that her inability to refuse others' requests was fueling the problem and that this inability likely related to her relationship with a rather critical, demanding parent. A brief psychodynamic therapy that focused on this issue proved very helpful to her and paved the way for successful problem solving later.

One way to understand how problem solving can complement other therapies is this: many forms of therapy (e.g., psychodynamic therapy, family therapy, and motivational interviewing, to name a few) help people recognize the need to change certain attitudes and behaviors. Problem solving helps people operationalize that change in real-life situations.

There is one particular area in child therapy, however, where problem solving appears to conflict with another form of therapy. In the area of childhood externalizing disorders, those practicing a therapy called "collaborative problem solving" (Greene, 2010) are sometimes in conflict with practitioners focusing on behavior modification. Collaborative problem solving is a family-focused therapy that advocates that parents plan ahead for situations where their child typically misbehaves and problem solve with the child to find better ways of managing these situations. The therapeutic goal is to help the child gradually learn effective ways of regulating upset feelings that result in misbehavior. Some practitioners of collaborative problem solving believe that having parents administer the consequences for child misbehavior (e.g., sending the child to her room for a time out) interferes with the child's ability to learn how to regulate upset feelings (Greene & Duncan, 2010).

Other child therapists (including myself) can see a role for both collaborative problem solving and behavior modification strategies. The former emphasizes parents managing the antecedents of misbehavior, while the latter emphasizes parents managing the consequences of mis-behavior, but both can be effective. For example, suppose the parents of a 9-year-old boy with ADHD report three main concerns:

1. Having his books gathered together for school in the morning before the school bus arrives.
2. Having him ask for food at the table rather than impulsively grabbing it.
3. Having him stop fighting with his younger sister after school while the mother is cooking dinner (when the father has not yet returned home from work), which happens a couple of times a week.

The first situation happens predictably every day, can be anticipated, and is largely within the boy's control. It is therefore very amenable to problem solving. The second situation is also predictable and daily, but the boy's degree of control may be limited because impulsivity is a symptom of ADHD. Nevertheless, problem solving may be worth a try. The third situation happens unpredictably, is not entirely within the boy's control (as the younger sister may sometimes provoke the fights), and happens at the end of a long day when the mother is coping with multiple demands without spousal support. In this situation, separating the children and sending both to their respective rooms seems considerably less complicated, and less likely to result in escalating family conflict and potential injuries, than any other solution. The parents may still want to engage in collaborative problem solving with the boy later to help him cope better with his sister's provocations, but in the heat of the moment this is unlikely to be effective.

In addition, time outs that occur with prior warnings can help some children learn to regulate upset feelings and tend to avoid undue attention to misbehavior. In one popular time out program, for example, the parent counts "That's one, that's two" and then times the child out only if the misbehavior is still present when the parent gets to "that's three" (Phelan, 2003). This consequence-focused approach motivates children to try to control their behavior when they hear "That's one" or "that's two," resulting in a gradually decreasing duration of misbehavior in response to upset feelings. By keeping the parent–child interaction brief and emotionally neutral, this system also avoids providing the child with extensive negative parental attention in response to misbehavior. Negative parental attention must be avoided, as it can inadvertently reinforce child misbehavior, making it worse. As in the example above, once the child is calm and cooperative, the antecedents of the problem can be addressed by using problem solving.

Similarly, problem solving can be readily combined with positive consequences. For example, anxious children often need to gradually face situations they fear in order to desensitize to the anxiety. To encourage this somewhat unpleasant process, therapists and parents may provide praise and other positive consequences when the child makes the effort to face a feared situation. However, planning how to face the feared situation (i.e., addressing the antecedents of the behavior) often includes problem solving with the child. The child may generate suggestions regarding small steps toward the feared situation (e.g., reading about the situation or seeing a video of the situation before going into it; going into the situation accompanied by a parent; going only partway into the situation, etc.), select from among several coping strategies to use in the situation (e.g., doing relaxed breathing, repeating reassuring statements, or bringing along a reassuring item from home), and even participate in selecting the positive consequence or reward.

In summary, many therapists use both problem solving and behavioral techniques when working with children and youth, but they place greater emphasis on one or the other at different times, depending on whether they want to address primarily the antecedents or primarily the consequences of the behavior in question.

Choosing the Order of Therapies

As discussed, there can be disadvantages to having the child participate in more than one therapy concurrently. Nevertheless, some children can benefit from two forms of psychotherapy if these are provided sequentially. Therefore, it is worth discussing when therapy focused on problem solving should be done first, and when second.

In the example of John, above, who had suffered the loss of his brother and severe burns in a house fire, a realistic problem needed to be addressed in order to allow his play therapy to proceed. This is one example of a situation where problem solving should be done first. Another common example relates to ensuring the feasibility of therapy. Consider the case of 15-year-old Samantha.

Samantha was a very good student but struggled with panic disorder and was motivated to work with a cognitive-behavioral therapist in her suburban community. Unfortunately, her mother was a single parent who had to work until late in the day to support her family, and the latest therapy appointment available was at 4:00 P.M. Thus, Samantha's mother could not drive her to appointments. Samantha's school day ended at 3:30 P.M., but the therapist's office was not within walking distance of her school, so she was not sure how to get to her therapy appointments.

Samantha's problem was defined as "finding a way to get to therapy appointments regularly at the end of the school day." Several alternatives were explored. First, Samantha and her mother explored bus routes and schedules in the area of Samantha's school. She could take the bus, but she would have to miss the last 20 minutes of class once a week to do so and was anxious about this, as she had never previously taken the bus independently. Second, Samantha considered cycling from school to the therapist's office. She would have to remember to bring her bicycle to school each day she had an appointment, though, and her mother was concerned about the risks of navigating a bicycle through traffic in the late afternoon. Third, Samantha's mother explored whether she could leave work early once a week and then work late another day to make up the time. The need to arrange coverage for her reception duties at her place of work, however, made this difficult. Fourth, Samantha and her mother asked if the therapist could see her in the evening. The therapist's own personal commitments precluded this, however. Fifth, Samantha considered asking one of her friends' parents to drive her to appointments, but she didn't like the idea of publicizing her need to see a therapist. Finally, Samantha and her mother considered looking for another therapist, but they decided against this because Samantha liked the therapist and there were no other therapists in their immediate area taking new clients. In short, none of the possible solutions was easy to implement, but several were feasible.

After weighing the pros and cons of each alternative, everyone agreed that taking the bus was the best option. Samantha's therapist provided an explanatory letter for her school, and Samantha was able to arrange for classmates' notes on the work she would miss. When evaluating the situation after a month, Samantha's therapist found that she had attended appointments consistently and on time, there was no deterioration in her school performance, and Samantha was pleased that she was able to use the bus independently.

Because problem solving involves planning ahead, it can also be introduced early in therapy when one can anticipate needing to implement certain strategies developed in that therapy or while waiting for therapeutic benefits to begin. For example, while children are learning strategies for coping with anxious situations, they can do some problem solving in anticipation of applying those strategies in their day-to-day lives. Similarly, changes resulting from behaviorally focused therapy for a child with ADHD may take time, but the child can still use problem solving to become more successful at getting out the door with all his school books in the mornings or to help remember to bring home his school day planner.

Problem solving can also be helpful when children and families face a mental health crisis but cannot immediately access a therapist. For example, psychiatrists seeing adolescents with suicidal thoughts in the emergency department often use problem solving to make a plan that ensures safety for a few days until the adolescent can begin psychotherapy and/or medical treatment. Of course, if the adolescent was planning to act on the suicidal thoughts, he or she would be admitted to hospital. If not, however, a problem-solving plan that reduces his or her risk of self-harm while awaiting treatment may be helpful. Locking up potentially dangerous items at home, arranging for additional supervision by family members, and encouraging the use of a telephone helpline if suicidal thoughts intensify might be some elements of that plan.

Problem solving should not be the first therapeutic intervention, however, when the child or adolescent is not motivated to make a change in behavior, lacks the skills needed to change the behavior, or when family interactions or other life circumstances are not conducive to successful problem solving. These issues were reviewed in Chapters 1 and 2, and must be addressed first before problem solving can succeed. Motivational problems are particularly relevant in situations where the current behavior represents a maladaptive coping strategy for regulating upset feelings. Substance abuse, eating disorders, acting-out behaviors, nonsuicidal self-injury (e.g., superficial cutting behaviors), and chronic avoidance behaviors all serve to regulate upset feelings in ways that are socially unacceptable and ultimately harmful to the child. These behaviors are difficult to address through problem solving, at least initially, because attempting to change them would engender additional distress for the child and sometimes for the family as well.

One situation where problem solving is sometimes attempted too quickly, for example, is in the treatment of chronic school avoidance. Typically these cases involve adolescents who initially avoided school because of an anxiety disorder or because of an unfortunate incident at school (e.g., being bullied by peers or being humiliated by a teacher) but who continued to avoid school for months or even years afterward. The avoidance of school becomes an entrenched behavior, family interactions begin to perpetuate the behavior, and the adolescent develops a new lifestyle involving ongoing school avoidance.

Well-meaning therapists and school personnel may use problem-solving techniques to formulate a plan for school reintegration with the teen and his or her parents. For example, various ways of ensuring transportation to school are explored, a schedule of initial classes to attend is made (with progressive increases in the number of classes attended each week), and a plan is formulated for helping the teen catch up on missed school work. The teen may or may not respond positively, but parents are often grateful for this plan and indicate a willingness to help implement it.

Unfortunately, no matter how expert the therapist or the school staff, the plan often does not work. Alternatively, it may work temporarily but the benefits disappear after the first weekend, as Mondays are almost always challenging for these teens. Repeated problem-solving attempts usually result in frustration on the part of the therapist and the school personnel, decreased cooperation by the families, and more school avoidance by the teen.

In this case, problem solving has been attempted in a situation where people are superficially cooperative but deeply fearful of change. Both the adolescent and the parent(s) have become accustomed to avoiding stress by avoiding changes in their daily routines and in their relationships with one another. School reentry by the adolescent threatens to expose him to the anxiety of facing a feared situation and of losing the comforts of home. The parent(s) are often anxious about exposing the adolescent to his anxiety, especially as some adolescents will make threats in response to parental requests to attend school (e.g., "I'll run away from home," "I'll kill myself rather than go to school"). Having the adolescent at home is also comforting to the parents in some cases (for example, offering companionship if the parent does not work outside the home or suffers from a physical disability or mental health problem). As long as the adolescent, the parent(s), or both harbor these anxieties and are comfortable with the adolescent's school avoidant lifestyle, the situation is unlikely to change.

In the long run, anxiety must be reduced and motivation to change increased in both the adolescent and the parent(s). Medication and CBT have both been found to be helpful for reducing anxiety in adolescents in this dilemma (Layne, Bernstein, Egan, & Kushner, 2003), and family-focused interventions are usually also needed to address parental anxiety and family interactions. Motivation to change can be addressed through motivational interviewing (e.g., identifying school-related goals for the teen; planning enjoyable activities for the stay-at-home parent) but usually also requires a change in the positive and negative consequences experienced when attending (vs. not attending) school. Addressing the specific circumstances that caused the absenteeism initially (e.g., bullying or conflict with teachers) reduces the potentially negative consequences of a return to school. Building the adolescent's skills for resuming a school-focused lifestyle (e.g., a good sleep regimen and effective study habits) and for dealing with peer reactions to prolonged absence increases the chances of school success (a positive consequence), as does an academic catch-up plan that is contingent on school attendance. Allowing the teen to suffer the natural consequences of school-avoidant behavior by, for example, having to deal with school failure and not being allowed to pursue favorite activities during the school day increases the negative consequences of remaining at home. Making the parent less available for interaction at home during the day reduces the positive consequences of the teen's staying there. Often more than one professional is needed so that therapy and skill building for the teen can occur with an individual he or she considers supportive, while behavioral, family, and school issues are addressed by another therapist.

Clearly, one cannot stop encouraging school attendance and planning for school return while waiting for these various interventions to work. However, change is unlikely to be dramatic until these contributing factors are addressed. Being realistic with school personnel about this fact in order to reduce frustration and discouragement is often helpful. One should not give up on problem solving with these adolescents, but recognize that they are unlikely to benefit until they and their families are both unequivocal about the need for consistent school attendance to resume and confident that this will occur.

COMBINING PROBLEM SOLVING
WITH MEDICATION

Problem solving and other psychotherapies are often combined with psychotropic medication in the treatment of children's mental health problems, and there is accumulating evidence that this combination may be helpful in many cases. Large randomized controlled trials done across several sites have confirmed the benefits of combining psychotherapy and medication in children with anxiety disorders (Walkup et al., 2008), obsessive–compulsive disorder (POTS Team, 2004), ADHD (March et al., 2000), and depression (Reinecke, Curry, & March, 2009). The studies vary in the degree to which the combination treatment benefits exceeded those of the psychotherapy or medication treatment alone, but generally the combination treatment was most helpful.

Not all children with mental health problems, however, need to take medication for these problems; children with mild or moderate symptoms often benefit from psychotherapy alone. Families often prefer to avoid having their children take medication unless it is deemed absolutely necessary. Furthermore, medication treatment in community settings is not always as helpful as medication treatment provided by experts (March et al., 2000). There are always attendant risks with medications, which must be weighed against their potential benefits in any given case. All of these considerations suggest that combining medication with psychotherapy should be done in a thoughtful way. Some key points to keep in mind when combining the two modalities are outlined in Table 8.1.

To begin, the need for the potential benefits of the medication to outweigh the risks suggests that medication should be reserved for children with severe impairment related to their mental health condition. Alleviating severe impairment allows the child's functioning to improve at home and at school, makes the child seem less deviant relative to peers (often improving self-esteem), and allows the child to resume a more normative developmental path. Such potential benefits usually offset the risks associated with a given medication. Children who are not severely impaired by their mental health condition may not derive the same degree of benefit from medication; so, the attendant risks of medication may or may not be worth taking in these children. A trial of psychotherapy alone may be worthwhile in these children to determine whether they can improve without the use of medication.

When medication and problem solving are combined, however, each may enhance the benefits of the other. Medication can make some children more amenable to problem solving. For example:

- Inattentive children who are given stimulant medication may become more focused, making it easier to engage them in problem solving.
- Children whose anxiety is reduced by medication may become calmer in therapy sessions, making it easier for them to learn coping strategies.
- Children whose depression is reduced by medication may become more hopeful about being able to solve problems and thus more motivated to engage in problem solving.
- Children whose aggressive behaviors are reduced by medication may suffer fewer school suspensions and other disruptive conse-

quences of aggressive behavior, enabling them to participate more consistently in therapy sessions.
• When their symptoms are reduced by medication, the children can often pursue a wider range of problem solutions than before (e.g., an anxious child may consider more solutions involving independent behavior than before; a withdrawn, depressed teen may consider more solutions involving social contact than before).

Conversely, problem solving can sometimes enhance the benefits of medication. For example:

• Problem solving can be used to help families evaluate the pros and cons of having the child take medication as well as the pros and cons of other therapeutic options, resulting in a more informed decision and greater commitment to that decision. This process can improve the chances of therapeutic success, regardless of what modalities are chosen.
• In families of severely impaired children who are reluctant to consider combining the technique with medication, a short trial of problem solving may demonstrate how much (or how little) benefit can be obtained with this modality alone, allowing for a more informed decision.
• Problem solving can be used to develop strategies for taking medication consistently, thereby improving adherence to the regimen.
• Successful problem solving may improve the child's functioning sufficiently that the child can manage with a lower dose of medication.
• Successful problem solving may improve the child's sense of self-efficacy, resulting in a more confident and independent child. Such self-efficacy may add to the benefits of medical treatment, particularly treatment for anxiety or depression.

Combining problem solving and psychotropic medication in children, however, does not always result in greater benefits than using either modality alone. Possible pitfalls of this combination include:

• Sometimes children and families assume that the child's problems must be very severe and not amenable to psychological intervention if medication is being recommended. This assumption may reduce their willingness to participate in problem solving. An educational approach that provides the evidence for all interventions being considered is often helpful in this case.

- Some medication side effects can adversely affect problem solving. For example, medications that are sedating or that result in cognitive slowing can make it harder for children to do problem solving successfully. Communicate with the prescribing physician about these side effects if they occur, as they may affect the child's school performance as well as his or her participation in therapy.

- If the prescribing physician and the therapist doing problem solving are the same person, medication side effects may adversely affect the client's level of trust in the therapeutic relationship.

- Sometimes medication reduces symptoms so dramatically that the therapist doing problem solving with the child struggles to find any problems to work on. In this case, negotiating a dosage reduction with the prescribing physician may be helpful to allow some symptoms (and thus some problems) to emerge. Alternatively, the child and family may decide to defer problem solving to a later date when they are able to reduce the child's reliance on medication.

- Sometimes children and families attribute improvements entirely to medication and therefore become unmotivated to do problem solving. Stabilizing medication first before starting problem solving may help avoid this problem. This practice clearly distinguishes benefits that result from medication from those that are attributable to problem solving.

- Sometimes children and families attribute improvements entirely to problem solving and therefore discontinue medication prematurely. Again, stabilizing medication first may help distinguish benefits resulting from each modality.

In summary, medication and psychotherapy focused on problem solving can interact in many ways, and not all of these are obvious. It is therefore well worth taking the time to explore with the children and their families how they feel about our treatment recommendations. As some of the points above illustrate, the psychological meanings attributed to medication and to psychotherapy can sometimes be just as important as their therapeutic effects. By understanding these meanings and offering clarification if needed, we improve the chances that the child will obtain the maximum benefit from any and all treatment modalities provided.

All of the points above also underscore the need for therapists and prescribing physicians to communicate regularly in order to deliver a coordinated treatment plan that provides the best care to the child and family. Communication that involves mutual respect for each other's areas of expertise is most likely to succeed. Often, a short telephone call or an e-mail is sufficient. If therapeutic obstacles are encountered, however, case conferences that enable the professionals to engage in problem solving together are sometimes helpful. As a psychiatrist, I have participated in such conferences at various times both as a prescribing physician and as a therapist. The ability to share frustrations with colleagues and then to formulate a plan that everyone contributes to and everyone is able to implement consistently is often invaluable. By working with our colleagues toward a common therapeutic goal, we avoid competing with them and derive the benefits of applying all of our resources in the best interests of the child.

Chapter 9

Problem Solving in Groups

Some people value child problem-solving groups for their capacity to treat many children at once, their cost effectiveness, and their ability to generate large numbers of ideas and solutions. Others would compare leading a child problem-solving group to "herding cats," because doing so requires that the leader keep many children focused on one issue for an extended period of time. The truth is probably somewhere in between these two points of view.

Child problem-solving groups have been found helpful in a variety of settings and for a variety of conditions. Groups with a mental health focus often incorporate problem solving as one of several skills taught and practiced by participants (Scapillato & Manassis, 2002). Problem-solving groups have also been used effectively in the management of chronic physical illnesses such as asthma (Pulgaron, Salamon, Patterson, & Barakat, 2010). Before any of these applications were developed, however, educators used group problem solving for years in their classrooms to teach academic skills (Kendall & Bartel, 1990). There are some differences in these approaches. For example, in mental health-focused groups, group members with similar difficulties typically decide on the specific problems to be solved, whereas in classroom settings teachers typically dictate the problems to be solved by the group. Nevertheless, these diverse applications speak to the versatility of group problem solving.

The potential advantages of child problem-solving groups over individual problem solving include universality (the comforting feeling of not being the only person with a given problem), peer support and encouragement, and the opportunity for productive brainstorming to generate large numbers of solutions. In order for these benefits to occur, however, therapists must invest considerable time and energy in managing group interactions so that the group remains focused on the problem-solving process. Structuring the group session, providing regular positive reinforcement for group participation, and occasionally attending to the individual needs of group members may also contribute to group success (Manassis et al., 2010). Selection of group members also requires some thought, as some groups of children have more difficulty working together than others.

Group composition, group rules, ways of establishing a well-functioning group, and managing group interactions in relation to the problem-solving steps will now be discussed, as these factors form the foundation of successful child problem-solving groups. Examples for different ages and different diagnostic groups will be included. The chapter concludes with considerations for dealing with challenging group members and group dynamics.

GROUP COMPOSITION

Grouping Children

Problem-solving groups in therapeutic settings typically consist of 4–10 children and one or two therapists. Working with fewer than four children limits the group's ability to generate multiple solutions, especially if one child is less active than the others or attends less consistently. Groups of more than 10 children are feasible (e.g., in classroom settings) but more difficult to manage. Both disruptive children and children who are difficult to engage in discussions require extra attention, and this is difficult to provide in groups that have more than 10 members.

Usually it is helpful to include children in a problem-solving group who have similar cognitive abilities and some diagnostic similarity. Children with similar cognitive abilities are able to work together at the same pace, reducing the chances of group members either feeling bored or being confused by the material. Limiting groups to a 3-year age span if possible, identifying any learning disabilities ahead of time, and conducting a pregroup interview for each child to ascertain oral and written communication ability are some ways of increasing the chances of a cognitively similar group. If running parent-focused problem-solving groups, including parents with a similar education level is usually helpful.

Diagnostic similarity makes it more likely that children will experience universality and find one another's problems interesting (as they are similar to their own), motivating them to work together. Alternatively, one can include children with different diagnoses but similar functional impairments. The latter is commonly done in social skills-focused groups. Some diagnoses, however, can have adverse effects on group interactions and should therefore be avoided or approached with caution. For example, adolescents who are all severely depressed will have difficulty engaging in group interactions. Conversely, children who all have severe ADHD will be difficult to manage in a problem-solving group, as they are unlikely to stay on task for any length of time. Both of these types of groups are feasible, however, if the most severe aspects of the psychopathology are treated ahead of time, for example, by providing appropriate psychotropic medication. One type of diagnostic group has been shown to be inadvisable: groups of children or adolescents with conduct disorder. In these groups, there is a high risk of group members learning antisocial behaviors from one another, even when therapists try to prevent it. Other interventions are available for these youngsters, but they involve family and social systems rather than focusing exclusively on the child (Woolgar & Scott, 2005).

Finally, there is some debate about the gender composition of problem-solving groups. Some therapists find there is more "common ground" among same-gender groups, while others argue that mixed-gender groups allow members to explore a wider range of interpersonal problems, as the perspectives of both boys and girls are represented. The participants' age and the focus of the group may also be relevant. For example, in classroom settings adolescent health programs are often separated by gender, but general science programs are not. There is some agreement, however, that one should avoid having only one boy in a group of mostly girls and one girl in a group of mostly boys. The discomfort of the "lone gender" participant often results in that child or adolescent dropping out of the group prematurely.

Group Therapists

If possible, it is helpful to run problem-solving groups with two therapists. These therapists need not be equally experienced. In fact, it is common in teaching institutions to pair an experienced therapist with a trainee. Whatever the pairing, an extra adult is useful in most cases to help lead the group and help manage group interactions. It is advisable for the two therapists to agree ahead of time on their respective roles. For example, one therapist may focus on the content of the group (i.e., teaching and leading the group through the problem-solving steps), while the other attends more to the group process (i.e., managing group interactions and challenging group members). Coordinating the work of two therapists does require a small amount of extra time: typically, a few minutes before each group session to plan their work and a few minutes after the group to "debrief" and decide on any change in their approach for the next session. It is well worth taking this time, though, as the sharing of therapists' observations about the group invariably enables them to learn from each other, regardless of whether or not one is training the other.

If only one therapist is available, then he or she must attend to both the content and the process of the group. Usually this results in some decreased attention to process, as most therapists naturally focus on content. When running a group alone, it is therefore helpful to ask oneself some basic questions about group process at the end of a session, in order to plan how to address these questions in the next session. These might include:

1. "Did any group member monopolize the discussion?"
2. "Did any group member not participate or participate very little?"
3. "Was any group member disruptive or disrespectful to other members or to me?"
4. "Did any group member make inappropriate comments suggesting a lack of understanding of the material or other issues?"
5. "Did I find any group member difficult or irritating for other reasons? Why?"
6. "Were there any problematic dyads within the group (either bothering each other or overly friendly)?"
7. "Was the mood of the group hopeful or anxious/pessimistic? Why?"
8. "Did group members seem interested and engaged in what we were doing? Why or why not?"
9. "Did the group stay on track and achieve the goals for this session? Why or why not?"

10. "Are there circumstances outside the group affecting one or more members' attitudes? (e.g., school exams, family conflicts, etc.)?"
11. "Was I hopeful, interested, and engaged in leading the group? Why or why not?"

Reflecting upon one's own reaction to the group or to particular group members (questions 5 and 11) is often an especially helpful source of clues to problematic group process.

GROUP RULES

Problem solving is a very structured process. Group members must be willing to follow that process step by step despite various distractions and potential interactions among them. In order for children and adolescents to cooperate with this process, it is important to establish some basic group rules in the initial session or first two sessions. It is very difficult to impose such rules later, when group members have already developed habitual ways of interacting that are inconsistent with those rules. A sample set of group rules is shown in Figure 9.1.

To avoid appearing like a punitive or dictatorial group leader, it is usually helpful to develop group rules collaboratively with all group members. Introduce the subject by saying something like "If we are

---

- We try to encourage and help one another with our problems.
- One person speaks at a time: we try not to interrupt each other.
- We finish discussing one problem before moving on to the next one.
- Different people have different points of view, so we try not to put down each other's ideas.
- If you are uncomfortable, it's OK to say, "I don't want to talk about that."
- What happens in the group stays in the group: we do not discuss other people's problems outside of the group.
- People who bother other people or break the rules are given a warning. If they don't stop, they have to sit out of the group for 5 minutes.
- It's important to come to the group every week: other people in the group depend on us.

FIGURE 9.1. Sample set of group rules.

going to work together to help one another with our problems, we need to make sure everyone feels safe and stays on track. What are some rules that might help us do that? I'll write down each rule once we all agree on it." A collaborative approach to rules is particularly important when working with adolescents, who often feel alienated and become disengaged when therapists try to tell them what to do.

Emphasizing the need to feel safe usually elicits several rules concerning mutual respect. These can include rules about trying to encourage and support one another, about respecting one another's confidentiality, about listening to one another's ideas nonjudgmentally, and about respecting each person's right to not discuss something he or she is not comfortable discussing. The need to respect confidentiality is particularly important in preadolescents, as younger children are prone to telling their family members about situations described by other group members, not realizing that the information might inadvertently get communicated back to that person. For example, a child once shared with a sibling the fact that another boy in the group was being raised by a single parent. That sibling saw the boy at school and asked, "So, what happened to your father?", reducing the boy to tears.

Emphasizing "staying on track" usually results in rules about taking turns when talking, finishing all the steps for one problem before moving on to the next one, and having a way to stop group members from distracting others or engaging in other misbehavior. Interestingly, when children or adolescents propose consequences for misbehavior, they are often more harsh than the 5-minute time out suggested in Figure 9.1. As a therapist, I have often had to modify proposed penalties so that the culprit was not hurt or badly humiliated and was able to continue contributing to the group.

One rule that therapists may need to spell out explicitly is the need for consistent attendance. Group participants often assume that if a session is missed they can catch up on the content the following week, and there is no other consequence to their absence. It is therefore important to describe how group members come to rely on one another for ideas, encouragement, and support. Thus, the absentee is not only limiting his or her own progress but also depriving other group members of his or her contribution. In fact, sometimes when a group member is absent, the rest of the group spends much of the session wondering about what happened to the missing member rather than attending to the task at hand.

If the group agrees, it may be helpful to share the group rules with the participants' parents as well, since these rules represent important treatment expectations. For example, the attendance rule definitely needs to be discussed with parents if they are responsible for bringing the child to the group. Parents may also be surprised to learn that their child may be disciplined for misbehavior in the group, though most accept this practice if it is spelled out at the beginning of the group sessions. For example, if a child continues to misbehave in the group despite a brief time out, parents may be contacted and asked to remove the child from the session. After the session concludes, they will be consulted about the best way to reintegrate their child into the group the following week. The confidentiality rule often reduces parents' natural tendency to ask their children to divulge details about group discussions or to try to obtain this information from the group therapist(s).

In order that parents not feel unduly excluded from the treatment process, however, it is usually helpful to describe to them the basic structure of problem solving. This allows parents to learn what their children are learning and to encourage its application outside the therapy room. Encouraging parents to voice any concerns that arise during the course of group sessions also fosters a sense of involvement and sometimes provides therapists with valuable information.

For example, Chris, a 12-year-old boy, was an engaged and popular member of a problem-solving group focused on social skills. His mother, however, reported that his grades were slipping, and he seemed apathetic about this fact. Chris's therapist suspected that, as his social skills had improved, he had begun spending more time with newly found friends and less time on homework. She decided to follow up on his mother's concern by prompting the group to think about the problem of finding time for both school and social activities. Eventually, Chris disclosed that he and his new friends had been skipping class and experimenting with marijuana in a secluded area behind the school. He liked his new friends but didn't like being pressured into smoking marijuana. The group supported Chris's attempts to resist peer pressure, an important social skill for all of them. Chris eventually returned to consistent class attendance and made new friends who did not use illicit drugs.

ESTABLISHING A WELL-FUNCTIONING GROUP

Before engaging in problem solving with a group of children, the therapist(s) need to establish a well-functioning group. Sometimes it is helpful to think of the group as an extra client who needs at least as much attention and assistance as any child in therapy.

Logistics

At the outset, the therapist(s) must ensure that the group has a private room that is available regularly for group meetings and must schedule meeting times when both therapists and the participating children are available. Weekly meetings are usually needed to ensure continuity from one session to the next. A board or flip chart is often helpful to keep track of the group's ideas and to illustrate problem-solving steps.

Rapport

Once group rules and expectations have been established (see above), initial sessions focus on building rapport among group members, setting goals for the group and for individual clients, getting into a structured routine for each session, and beginning to learn the problem-solving steps. Having each group member share something interesting about him- or herself is a common exercise for starting to develop rapport. Asking each child his or her favorite game, favorite movie, or favorite activity can also be used to break the ice. Children should not be pressured to disclose more than they are comfortable telling, however, as some do require several sessions to warm up to the group situation. If the therapist(s) participates in the exercise, this can make him or her appear more human and less threatening, particularly to anxious group members. Once each member has spoken, the therapist(s) can summarize the information and point out common themes (e.g., "Nancy, Joe, and Shakil all like soccer, and Trevor and Sarah both play guitar"). Knowing that they have certain interests or activities in common increases children's sense of belonging to a group and their trust of other group members.

In addition to trusting one another, group members must also learn to trust their therapist(s). Providing a predictable structure for each group session reduces group members' anxiety and increases trust in the therapist(s) as well as helping to keep the group focused. In problem-solving groups, this structure usually includes updates on solutions tried the preceding week, introducing a new topic for the session, problem-solving exercises related to that topic, deciding what solutions will be implemented in the week to come, and a brief social time at the end (often accompanied by a light snack). Asking about children's individual goals within the group and asking for feedback at the end of each session lends further credibility to the therapists, showing that they are sincere in their concern for each group member.

Adolescents may require some additional strategies to ensure their engagement in the group. Therapists must still structure the group sessions so that they can be productive, but they must also respect adolescents' increasing need for autonomy and increasing cognitive sophistication. To respect autonomy, sessions are typically less didactic than with younger children, and group members are allowed to make some choices about the content of sessions. A greater emphasis on the confidentiality of group information is also needed in adolescents than in younger children. Consistent with increased cognitive sophistication, adolescents need to be provided with a clear rationale as to how the group and the problem-solving process are thought to be helpful. Therapists must be prepared to answer pointed questions about this rationale and should welcome a degree of skepticism among group members. Rather than trying to "sell" the merits of the group, therapists may do better emphasizing to adolescents that they will get out of the group what they put into it. In other words, positive change results from a collaborative process within the group, which can only happen when members participate. Once engaged in the group, however, adolescents can use this type of treatment very effectively. Because it mirrors their usual social milieu, adolescents are able to use the group as a safe forum for social problem solving, use peers in the group as positive role models, and gain confidence by implementing their new solutions with minimal assistance from adults (Scapillato & Manassis, 2002).

From Dictatorship to Democracy

Successful problem-solving groups gradually change from being therapist-led to becoming forums for group members to solve problems autonomously. Thus, metaphorically, the group changes from a dictatorship to a democracy. The emphasis on group rules, session structure, and teaching problem-solving steps is important in the beginning to teach children and adolescents to work together in a focused, productive way. It is much easier to adjust an overly strict initial approach by eventually relaxing certain rules than to try to impose new rules on a disorganized group after several sessions.

As in individual work, problem-solving steps are taught and then applied to situations children are struggling with in their lives. To encourage increasing group autonomy and a decreasing focus on the therapist, therapists can begin by modeling problem-solving steps and helping the group solve hypothetical problems before moving on to encouraging and coaching the group to solve problems they have generated themselves and prompting group members to help one another solve problems. Finally, if the group dynamics develop as desired, therapists will be praising and encouraging independent group problem solving.

Prompting group members to help one another solve problems is sometimes challenging, but a few leading questions may help. These may include one or more of the following, first with respect to generating alternative solutions:

- "What do other people in the group think about that?"
- "Has anyone in the group ever faced a similar situation? What did you do?"
- "What would you do [looking at another group member] in that situation?"
- "Can anyone help [group member] with that dilemma?"
- "Let's see how many ideas we can come up with for that situation. I'll keep track. Who has one?"

And then with respect to evaluating and selecting solutions:

- "What an interesting idea; how do people think that would work?"
- "Let's take a moment to look at that idea. Do people think it would work or not? Why? Why not?"
- "What would happen if [group member] did that?"
- "Sounds like most people would favor this idea. Is that right? Any objections?"
- "Is everyone comfortable with that plan?"

GROUP DYNAMICS
AND THE PROBLEM-SOLVING STEPS

Each of the problem-solving steps makes different demands on the group, but from the therapist's point of view they break down into two group management challenges: keeping the group focused and encouraging the group to generate multiple ideas (called brainstorming). Selecting a problem to solve, selecting a solution to implement, trying it out, and evaluating the results are all steps that require the group to remain focused. Generating possible problems to be discussed, generating alternative solutions for a given problem, and "fine-tuning," or suggesting additional solutions if the one tried doesn't work, are all steps that require the group to generate multiple ideas.

Much of the discussion so far in this chapter has focused on establishing a focused, productive group and ensuring that participants are engaged enough to contribute to the group. Often members of groups with this foundation are motivated to help one another and therefore generate ideas easily.

Difficulties in generating ideas can relate to the characteristics of group participants, problematic group interactions, or the nature of the problem being discussed. Sometimes a number of group members are shy or inhibited and need encouragement to contribute ideas (see below). Group interactions that inhibit everyone's desire to brainstorm include previous negative or judgmental responses to certain ideas and a belief that generating many ideas will prolong the problem-solving process and thus delay social or snack time. Therapists can mention each of these possibilities, see if they reflect the group's concerns, and then address them if needed. Finally, the nature of the problem being discussed may make it difficult for the group to generate alternative ideas. Refer back to Chapter 3 to review the characteristics of problems that are amenable to a problem-solving approach. Sometimes, even with an appropriate choice of problem, however, the group may struggle to find alternative solutions. Consider the example of Muniya.

Muniya was a 10-year-old girl in a problem-solving group who described eating lunch at school. Her lunch, though lovingly prepared by her mother, was different from the lunches all of the other children ate. Muniya was embarrassed about eating a lunch that reflected her ethnic background, and she had been teased about her food more than a few times. At the same time, she did not want to criticize her mother's food and was anxious about asking her mother for a different type of lunch. Muniya wanted to be able to eat lunch without experiencing teasing or embarrassment—but also without offending her mother.

In trying to generate alternative solutions for this dilemma, the group was stumped. None of the other children had experienced this sort of problem. "My mom sometimes makes bologna sandwiches, which I hate, but none of the other kids care," volunteered one girl in the group, trying to be helpful. Then there was silence in the room.

The therapist wisely decided to broaden the discussion in this case, exploring the possibility that others had experienced situations that were similar, though not identical, to Muniya's. She said to the group, "We may not all eat special foods for lunch, but I'll bet there are other reasons people sometimes find lunchtime at school difficult or embarrassing. Can anyone think of any?"

Within a few minutes, the group members had thought of several embarrassing lunchtime situations. One child wore special braces that needed to be removed before each meal, eliciting negative comments from other children. Another had a food allergy and therefore couldn't trade lunches with other children (a common practice at his school). Another child mentioned a friend who couldn't buy a snack with lunch (as most children at her school did) because the friend's family didn't have much money. Another child's friend had to go to the office during lunch hour to be given medication. Next, the therapist asked how the children dealt with these situations and then applied the same solutions to Muniya's dilemma. Their ideas included briefly explaining the reason for one's "different" lunch routine, seeing the difference as interesting rather than problematic, thinking of an assertive comeback in the event of teasing, and involving an adult if teasing persisted. By the end of the discussion, Muniya not only had some helpful ideas to address her dilemma, but she also felt she had a lot in common with the rest of the group.

CHALLENGING GROUP MEMBERS AND GROUP INTERACTIONS

Sometimes despite the therapist's best efforts to maintain a focus on problem solving and to manage group interactions, certain group members pose therapeutic challenges. These usually relate to either the quantity or quality of the member's participation in the group. Group members who participate very little are just as challenging as those who monopolize the group. Inappropriate forms of group participation pose a further challenge.

Members Who Participate Too Little

Low levels of group participation can relate to the child's temperament, psychological or cognitive problems, lack of motivation, the actions of other group members, or a combination of these factors. For example, it is common for temperamentally shy or inhibited children to appear disengaged because they do not volunteer many ideas in a group. However, other group members may be behaving in ways that the inhibited child finds intimidating; or they may assume that the inhibited child has nothing to contribute since he or she has not joined the discussion. When people do not join a discussion within the first 5 minutes, other participants often assume that they do not intend to do so or have nothing to say. Children who appear withdrawn because of depressive symptoms may face similar difficulties. Unless this problem is addressed, the inhibited or depressed child may feel increasingly alienated from the rest of the group and be at risk of dropping out.

An astute therapist, however, will recognize this problem and attempt to elicit the child's participation. This must be done in a sensitive manner, though, as some children are embarrassed if the therapist "puts them on the spot" by asking a direct question. If the therapist is aware of the child's main issues and goals, participation can be prompted by saying, "We haven't talked about X [child's issue] for a while. Let's spend a few minutes coming up with some ideas about that." Children are more likely to participate if the topic is relevant to their needs. Alternatively, the therapist can ask for input without singling out the child by, for example, saying, "Any ideas from this side of the room?" or "Does anyone else in the group have an idea?" Silence can even be reframed positively by saying, "[Child's name], you've been listening to this discussion very patiently. I'd like to give you a chance to say something if you wish. Do you have any thoughts about this topic?" With this reassuring invitation, some children are able to contribute an idea, which the therapist can then praise. If not, the child will at least feel obliged to say "No" or "I don't have anything to add." Having spoken once in this context, the child is then more likely to be invited to speak by other group members subsequently. If none of these approaches seems to be working, have a cotherapist or another group member engage the child in conversation one on one. Doing so is often a helpful step toward the child's eventual group participation.

Children who do not engage in group discussions owing to a lack of motivation usually require a different approach. These children typically indicate their lack of interest through body language or avoiding eye contact. They may also make disparaging remarks at the beginning or end of the group such as "Here we go again (sigh)," or "Well, that was a waste of time." These children do not participate in group discussions because they are doubtful that the group will provide them with anything of value. They may also feel disconnected from other group members.

Eliciting goals from each group member at the outset (see above) and reflecting back on these goals periodically is sometimes helpful for these children. The therapist can then, for example, invite the group to focus on solving a problem relevant to the disengaged member's main goal. Alternatively, exercises that foster connections between group members are sometimes helpful. Partnering the disengaged child with a more engaged "buddy" or assigning the disengaged child tasks that are helpful to others in the group are examples of this approach.

Children who are cognitively at a different level than the rest of the group may also benefit from these motivating strategies. Cognitively advanced children may be bored by the slow pace of the group, and cognitively limited children may be confused and therefore feel out of step with the rest of the group. In addition, these children may benefit from individualized attention (from a cotherapist, if available) to better meet their needs. Therapists must, however, carefully balance the need for individual attention to cognitive differences with the need to allow the child to be a contributing, valued member of the group. One-on-one time should therefore be provided only when necessary.

Members Who Dominate

At the opposite end of the spectrum from the low-participation group member is the member who dominates the group. At first glance, this child's behavior may not appear problematic. After all, a group member who contributes significantly to the discussion and even sometimes leads it seems like a very helpful participant. When a group member begins to dominate conversation, however, others can find it difficult to participate and may even feel excluded from the work of the group. Some dominant group members also try to ingratiate themselves with the group leader(s), behaving almost like cotherapists. Other children usually respond to this behavior with resentment, for example calling the dominant member a "teacher's pet," "leader's favorite," or other unflattering term. Ingratiating children also like to give others advice, sometimes reducing their opportunities to discuss their own problems.

Therefore, it is important for therapists to set limits on children who tend to dominate a group. To limit dominating behavior, therapists can redirect the focus of the group to other members by saying, for example, "That's a really interesting idea, but we haven't heard from [child X] and [child Y] yet. Let's hear what they have to say." Alternatively, therapists can redirect the focus of the group to the task at hand by saying, "We need to wrap up our discussion of problem X soon; so, let's see if there are other ideas about that problem." The latter approach is particularly helpful if the dominating member is making comments that distract from the task at hand. The ingratiating child, on the other hand, sometimes benefits from a focus on his or her own specific problem. "I recall you've been struggling with X" might be a way to introduce the subject. This remark clearly places the child in the role of group member rather than cotherapist and ensures that his or her needs are addressed.

Inappropriate Forms of Participation

Some group members neither dominate nor withdraw from group interactions but, rather, participate in inappropriate ways. Children who distract other group members from the problem-solving process can be particularly challenging. Sometimes children with ADHD exhibit this behavior, although unmotivated or attention-seeking children may also do so. Some common distracting behaviors include making irrelevant or goofy remarks, prodding or teasing others, talking out of turn, exhibiting odd facial expressions or gestures, or drawing attention to objects in the room that are unrelated to the discussion. Moreover, when one group member begins to exhibit distracting behaviors, others often follow suit, resulting in a chaotic group that is difficult to manage.

Minor distracting or silly behavior sometimes diminishes if it is ignored. However, therapists may need to set limits for repeat offenders. To limit distracting behaviors, therapists can begin by redirecting the focus of the group to other members, as outlined above for dominating behaviors. In addition, however, therapists may need to reiterate group rules and seat certain group members apart from one another to avoid a chaotic group. Repeated distracting behavior is clearly against the rules, as it bothers others and interferes with the work of the group; so, it usually merits a brief time out apart from the rest of the group. Usually the child is seated in a chair in the corner of the room for 5 minutes before being allowed to rejoin the group. If this is done in a calm matter-of-fact way, the child often settles down. If misbehavior continues, the child's caregiver may be contacted, as noted earlier in the chapter. Also, therapists in many groups provide children with a snack or other small reward for successfully completing the group's work at the end of the session. In this case, group members can be reminded that snack time is contingent on finishing their work. This reminder reduces the chances that they will emulate the distracting group member and may even result in other members scolding the offender or otherwise trying to limit his or her misbehavior.

Finally, some group members exhibit behaviors that are inappropriate or that others consider strange. Discussing things in the group that are not consistent with the focus of the group, or trying to discuss things outside the group (e.g., with the therapist in the hallway) that clearly belong in the group are common examples of inappropriate behavior. Usually the child exhibiting such behavior can be gently redirected to good effect. If several children in the group behave this way, a clear rule about what types of issues are discussed in the group and about therapist contact outside the group may be needed. Similarly, rules about using expletives or other inappropriate language are sometimes needed. Odd or strange behaviors rarely occur in groups when children are carefully assessed for group suitability, but they do happen occasionally. For example, a child may exhibit inappropriate sexualized behaviors or innuendos in the group. During the group session the therapist(s) must limit such behaviors, as they are normally disturbing to other group members. Afterward, however, the therapist has a responsibility to further assess the child and contact appropriate child protective services if there is indeed a suspicion of abuse.

Problematic Interactions among Members

Interactions between certain group members can also be challenging to manage. Members who dislike each other can clearly be difficult, but members who are especially fond of each other can also pose challenges. Having clear group rules usually minimizes open hostility between members, but children have other ways of communicating anger or contempt for one another. Be alert for children who roll their eyes or chuckle when another member speaks, use sarcasm or make disparaging remarks about others' ideas, or simply ignore another group member's contributions. If two members dislike each other but do not involve others in the group, the therapist can address the situation like a parent addresses sibling rivalry: by positively reinforcing each member for his or her unique contributions and trying not to attend more to one than the other. If, on the other hand, one member tries to ally the rest of the group against another member, the therapist must intervene more decisively. Victimization of one group member by other members cannot be permitted; so, the therapist must support and protect the excluded child. In this case, it is also appropriate to devote at least one group session to an empathic discussion of bullying and victimization, even if this subject is not the main focus of the group. Most children who bully have also had the experience of being victimized and are able recognize the harmfulness of this type of behavior.

Group members who are especially fond of each other can distract the group from its work, and they sometimes miss opportunities to learn from the group because of their preoccupation with each other. In younger children, this behavior often manifests as two members chatting together apart from the rest of the group. In adolescents, the interaction may go beyond chatting to include romantic words or gestures. If this type of behavior occurs occasionally, the therapist can use the strategies described above for distracting behaviors, including a change in the seating arrangement (i.e. seating the "couple" apart from each other). If the behavior becomes more frequent or intense, a discussion with the two members outside the group may be needed. Rather than simply chiding them for misbehavior, it may be helpful to also point out the effects on other group members (e.g., "How would you feel if you saw two other people in the group carrying on like this?"), the fact that they are losing opportunities to work on their presenting issues in the group, and the time-limited nature of the group. Friendships that become intense in a time-limited group and may not be sustainable afterward can result in unhappiness and (if romantic) heartbreak.

Problematic Group Interaction Patterns

Sometimes patterns of interaction within the whole group require the therapist's attention. Inconsistent attendance, a very quiet group, a group that expresses a lot of pessimism, or a very boisterous group can all be a cause for concern. Problems with attendance or participation can suggest a lack of confidence in the group's potential for being helpful or a lack of cohesion within the group. Activities focused on engaging group members and on building cohesion are often helpful. For example, therapists can illustrate concepts by using exercises that require everyone to participate cooperatively, such as having each child take a turn contributing to a group drawing or the group's list of ideas. Group role plays to rehearse new solutions can also be very engaging. Having each child work with a partner and then both present their ideas to the larger group may also help children feel connected to their peers. Having a few minutes of social time at the end of the group as a reward for working together effectively can also improve children's motivation to participate.

Pessimistic groups may offer group members a lot of mutual support by allowing for frequent commiseration, but they tend to produce few alternative solutions to problems. If members are pessimistic about the possibility of improving their lives, their motivation to problem-solve may be limited. Challenging the pessimism too strongly, however, can give children the impression that the therapist is ignoring or invalidating their feelings. A combination of empathy and redirection is most helpful. The therapist can say, for example, "It's good to know that most of you are struggling with this issue, because it's an important [or difficult or tricky] one, but let's see if we can come up with some ideas on how to deal with it." Then, positively reinforce any relevant ideas and summarize them frequently to show group members what they are accomplishing. If nobody volunteers, the therapist can propose an idea or two and ask for the group's feedback on why it would or wouldn't work. Another strategy is for the therapist to amplify the group's pessimism to an unrealistic degree (e.g., by saying, "I'm sure this would be completely impossible … "), prompting one or more group members to correct him or her and shift to a more realistic (and therefore less pessimistic) perspective.

Children in boisterous groups may enjoy interacting with one another but accomplish little because their interactions are not focused on the problem-solving process. They may also be disrespectful or challenge the therapist's control over the group. In this case, it is tempting to simply refer back to the group rules and punish the worst offenders. Sometimes this approach reestablishes a more orderly group process, but at other times it may alienate the group from the therapist. For example, toward the end of a session most children in the group may be getting restless and distracted. In this case, having a break, changing seats, having children stand or walk across the room as they contribute ideas, or even inviting one of the children to lead a group problem-solving exercise may be helpful. These strategies can dissipate some of the group's energy in ways that do not interfere with the work of the group or make the therapist appear unduly punitive.

Finally, unexpected crises in the lives of group members can be challenging for the therapist to manage. Examples include group members who encounter a major life event such as a serious illness or death in the family, group members who become acutely suicidal, or group members who become too disturbed to continue participating in the group. In most cases, children will respond with sympathy for the affected group member and worry about his or her well-being. Parents may express concerns about contagion in the group (e.g., the idea that their child could become suicidal after hearing another child express suicidal thoughts), and therefore they need reassurance that there is a very low risk of this happening. The therapist's primary responsibility is to ensure safety for the affected group member, using emergency resources if needed—

regardless of any confidentiality concerns. Children in the group usually understand the reasons for this approach and are glad that an adult is taking charge of the situation. They may, however, also need a brief explanation of what has happened and the opportunity to discuss their questions and concerns about the affected group member. If the affected member is unable to return to the group, updates on his or her progress are also important to provide, to reassure group members so that they can continue working together effectively.

Chapter 10

Problem Solving
with Parents and Families

$\mathbf{I}$t has been said that every unhappy family is unhappy in its own way (Tolstoy, 1877/1977). As someone who has tried to apply problem solving with parents and with families, I have often found this to be true. In order to be helpful to families, therapists need to understand the norms and values they hold dear and the communication patterns they typically follow. Family values will determine what problems are important to solve in a particular family, and communication patterns give clues as to how to approach the problem-solving process with that family.

Therefore, this chapter focuses less on the steps of problem solving than on parent and family characteristics that are important to ensure that problem solving is successful. The key ideas about each problem-solving step are identical whether one is working with children, adolescents, parents, groups, or families. Thus, when working with parents or families, the chapters pertaining to these steps should be read in addition to this one.

PARENT-FOCUSED PROBLEM SOLVING

The need to gain parents' consent and approval for new solutions has already been discussed in previous chapters. In some situations, however, it is important for parents to participate actively in implementing new solutions in order for problem solving to succeed or to result in lasting benefits. In these situations, therapists work directly with parents and engage in parent-focused problem solving. The most obvious role for parent-focused problem solving is in the treatment of young children, who are highly dependent on their parents to develop new behaviors. Indeed, there is evidence that parental coaching of new behaviors is more crucial to the successful treatment of younger children than older children (Barrett, Dadds, & Rapee, 1996). Parent-focused problem solving can also be employed in situations where children are not motivated to try new behaviors without parental encouragement, most commonly externalizing problems (e.g., oppositional behavior or conduct problems). Problem-solving programs focused on parents have been shown to be highly effective in these cases as well (Greene, 2010; Webster-Stratton, Reid, & Hammond, 2004).

Even when children are motivated to try new behaviors, parents can still play important roles, including encouraging children to practice new behaviors in different settings and facilitating children's independent problem solving. For example, an anxious child may make considerable progress in using new coping strategies in the therapist's office but find it difficult to use these same strategies outside of the office. The ability to generalize new strategies to real-world situations outside of the office often requires support from parents. Thus, a child with a fear of elevators may ride calmly up and down the hospital elevator at the end of therapy but still need parental support to manage the same behavior in an apartment building. Involving parents in such exposure exercises has been found to increase the benefits of evidence-based treatments for childhood anxiety (Manassis, 2005; Mendlowitz et al., 1999), and successful parental involvement often includes considerable planning and problem solving.

Children's development of independent problem-solving skills may also require parental support. For example, if a child wants to learn to sleep alone in his or her own bed without fear and the parent asks, "What could we do differently at bedtime?", the child may respond with a blank stare. However, if the parent says, "Let's put a dime on the table for every idea we can come up with to make bedtime less scary!", the child may rise to the challenge and brainstorm with the parent effectively. Then the parent can help the child evaluate which ideas are most likely to be feasible and helpful and thus positively reinforce the child's willingness to try these. In this case, the parent is guiding the child through the problem-solving steps in a manner likely to produce a successful outcome, thus increasing the chances of the child's being willing and able to problem-solve independently later on. Numerous benefits have been associated with children's ability to problem-solve independently, including increased confidence, enhanced cognitive development through active learning, and the gradual development of autonomous behaviors consistent with the child's abilities (reviewed in Brooks & Goldstein, 2001). The ability to engage in independent problem solving is also considered an important aspect of children's resilience (the ability to cope effectively with adversity) (Brooks & Goldstein, 2001).

Therapeutic Work with Parents

In order for parents to effectively problem-solve the management of their children's behavior, to support their children's use of new behaviors in different settings, and to gradually facilitate their children's independent use of problem solving, therapists must discuss these outcomes as explicit goals of therapy. Parents lead busy lives and are often glad to drop off their child at the therapist's office, hoping that he or she is able to change the child's behavior for the better. The importance of parents' own work with the child must be emphasized as the therapist guides parental efforts. Children's desire to please their parents, parents' empathy and desire to help their children, parents' familiarity with what rewards or consequences their children find motivating, and the considerable time parents spend with their children daily all speak to the high potential impact of parents on child behavior. Spelling out these facts to parents often encourages them, especially in situations where parents feel relatively helpless in the face of their children's problems.

Parents of teens may be particularly doubtful about their own abilities to influence their adolescents' behavior. For these parents, it may be helpful to emphasize that their teens see them as role models even when they do not readily acknowledge this fact. In other words, many adolescents do not do as their parents say, but they may still do as their parents do. Moreover, parents can still insist on certain behavioral standards as long as the teen is living at home. They may not be able to force their adolescent to perform or avoid a particular behavior, but they can reward or discourage it by, for example, providing an extra privilege or not providing an allowance.

More convincing than facts, however, are the results of successful problem solving. Meet with one or both parents regularly, and focus on a specific problem to solve. Then, have them implement a new solution with the child and report back the next week on the result. Seeing their efforts make a difference builds parents' confidence and sets the stage for gradually turning over leadership of the problem solving process to them. Later, once parents are successful problem-solvers, they can guide their children to develop the same skill set.

Challenges in Problem Solving with Parents

Once parents understand the important impact they can have on their children's behavior, many are motivated to begin problem solving. As with group counseling (see Chapter 9), there are two common challenges in problem solving with parents: keeping them focused and encouraging them to generate multiple ideas. Selecting a problem to solve, selecting a solution to implement, trying it out, and evaluating the result are all steps that require focused attention. Generating possible problems to be discussed, generating alternative solutions for a given problem, and "fine-tuning," or suggesting additional solutions if the one tried doesn't work, are all steps that require parents to generate multiple ideas. A further challenge in working with parents and families is that they have a history together, and therefore have certain patterns of interaction that may help or hinder the problem-solving process (discussed further in the "Family-Focused Problem Solving" section below).

Focusing on one problem can be disconcerting for some parents, who may feel that their children have many behaviors that need to change and who are impatient to see results. If this is the case, emphasize that the goal of working together is not just to solve problems but to learn an *approach* to problem solving so that this skill can be applied to issues arising throughout their child's development. Focusing on one problem can also be difficult for families of inattentive children. In these families, the child's behavior may result in a somewhat chaotic home environment, and (given the genetic link to their children) the parents may be somewhat inattentive themselves.

Selecting a new solution to try may be difficult if the parents disagree. Often this occurs when one parent sees the child's behavior as willful and perhaps deserving of punishment while the other sympathizes with the child. In this case, a skillful therapist will help the parents to find a "middle ground" by emphasizing which solutions could best help the child's behavior to change. Children rarely change their behavior when parents become angry, nor are they likely to change it when parents sympathize. A firm but emotionally neutral response that both parents can agree upon is usually most effective, but it can take several sessions for parents to develop such a response. For example, if a child is anxious about sleeping independently, one parent may sympathize if the child describes noises in the house that sound like burglars and allow the child to come to the parents' room under these circumstances while the other parent may exclaim, "We have a security system, for Pete's sake! Don't be silly! Go back to your room." It may be difficult for these parents to agree on a solution that both can implement consistently, given their differing perspectives. In order for the child to cope with his or her fear, however, the parents must develop a response that is empathic and calm and that encourages progress toward independent sleep. One response fitting this description would be allowing the child to call out but remain in his or her room when afraid, having a parent consistently go to the child and provide calm, brief reassurance in response, and charting these parental "visits" the next morning. Then, the child can be positively reinforced for decreasing their frequency.

Consistent implementation of new solutions can be difficult for parents with many competing priorities. It is common for parents to skim through numerous parenting guides but not apply any of the ideas they have read to their child. Even when committed to a new idea, parents may forget to apply it in the midst of a busy workweek or apply it inconsistently. Writing down the new solution and everyone's role in it is often helpful, especially if this information is then posted in a prominent location (e.g., on the refrigerator or family bulletin board). Most families also need to set a consistent time for following up and evaluating results. A weekly parent meeting or family meeting on the same day at the same time increases the chances of regular follow-up.

Generating alternative solutions can pose several difficulties for parents. Some parents are anxious about coming up with the "wrong" solution, and so they look to the therapist to tell them what to do rather than brainstorming. Emphasize for these parents that, regardless of the outcome of the new solution, something will be learned from the exercise. In fact, sometimes more will be learned if the solution doesn't work very well than if it does. All parents make mistakes occasionally, and, as long as the parents' behavior is not abusive, these mistakes usually do not result in long-term damage to their children.

Some parents do not have this anxiety but nevertheless struggle with generating alternatives. In this case, ask some leading questions such as "Some parents have told me they tried X. Do you think that might work at your house?" or "What have your friends/relatives suggested?" or "What would happen if you did Y?" or "What would you suggest to your neighbor if her child had this problem?" Many of these questions are phrased in terms of other people or other people's children.

This is deliberate, as parents often find it less threatening to talk about others' families or others' opinions rather than their own.

Another difficulty is that some parents always seem to generate the same type of alternative. This is common in families where one or both parents struggle with anxiety or depression themselves. Anxious parents tend to think of solutions that involve avoidance of anxiety-provoking situations for themselves and their children (Barrett, Rapee, Dadds, & Ryan, 1996). For example, a child may be anxious about presenting his or her project in front of the class. The parent, in an effort to help, may offer to talk to the teacher about having the child graded based on written work alone. The result (avoidance of presentations) alleviates the child's distress in the short term but perpetuates his or her performance anxiety in the long term. Depressed parents may have difficulty believing that their child can change his or her behavior at all or may feel hopeless about ever understanding the reasons for the child's behavior. "If you were in your child's situation, what would you want the adults around you to say?" is sometimes a good question for these parents. By putting themselves in their children's shoes, these parents can sometimes begin to appreciate reasons for their children's behaviors and see potential solutions where none seemed to exist before. This approach is described in more detail in the book *Helping Your Teenager Beat Depression* (Manassis & Levac, 2004).

Finally, some parents cannot or should not be asked to engage in problem solving with respect to their children's behavior until they have undergone other types of counseling. Parents who have severe untreated mental health problems clearly fit this category. Therapists should also, however, be cautious when working with parents who may appear quite rational in the initial interview but may suffer from undiagnosed personality disorders that affect their parenting. Often such problems are revealed only when the parent begins to problem-solve and the new solutions generated reflect either a consistent lack of empathy for the child or developmentally inappropriate expectations of the child. If parents are allowed to implement these types of solutions, the therapist may be inadvertently contributing to behavior that is psychologically harmful or (in some cases) frankly abusive to the child.

For example, a young mother appeared puzzled as she told the therapist, "I don't know why Brad is so upset. I told him if he improved his marks I would reward him, like we discussed." "What reward did you suggest?" the therapist asked. "I told him he could have a chocolate cake for his birthday next week," she replied. "Does Brad really like chocolate cake?" the therapist inquired. "It's not his favorite, but his brother and sister both like it, and who wouldn't be grateful for a chocolate cake?" she responded. She simply couldn't understand why her son would be upset about being offered his siblings' favorite treat as a reward, showing a clear lack of empathy.

In this case, the therapist could encourage the mother to repeatedly "put herself in her son's shoes" (see above) when problem solving. Some parents can develop empathy for their children in response to such exercises. Those who cannot often need further mental health evaluation themselves.

Similarly, developmentally inappropriate expectations can be a "red flag" for parental personality problems and possible risk of abusive behavior toward the child. This is particularly concerning when children are expected to behave in an adult-like manner or in a manner that does not respect the psychological boundary between parent and child. For example, one divorced father reported, "Amy is so helpful. She listens to me at the end of a long day at work the way her mother never did. We always enjoy those talks while watching the ballgame." It's possible that this comment reflects some harmless father–daughter bonding, but the fact that the father is comparing his daughter to his ex-wife, using her as a confidante (usually an adult role), and speaking for his daughter when saying "*We* always enjoy … " (suggesting a poor psychological boundary between parent and child), should alert the therapist to the possible risk of sexual abuse. Additional inquiries about the nature of their relationship should be undertaken to clarify this risk—before doing any further therapeutic work with this father. It is common, however, for parents who are single, divorced, or widowed to confide in their children more so than those in two-parent households. Thus, the father's report does not warrant an accusation of abuse, merely further inquiries.

Helping Parents to Encourage Child Problem Solving

Once parents are able to engage in problem solving with the therapist, their next challenge is to help promote problem-solving skills in their children. Young children may need considerable help with problem solving and may not be able to undertake all the steps on their own at first. Nevertheless, even children in their early school years can be given choices about the foods they eat, the clothes they wear, the activities they would like to pursue after school or on weekends, and other day-to-day events. Later, they can be asked to give reasons for their choices (practicing evaluating alternatives to make selections) and then asked to reflect upon the outcome of the choice. "What are some things you could do in this situation?" or "What are your choices here?" are good questions to prompt children to think about alternatives. By the preteen years, many children can begin to put the various problem-solving steps together with their parents' help. Having practiced problem solving with parental help as children, they can then problem-solve independently by adolescence.

Parents of adolescents who did not engage in any problem solving as children have not necessarily "missed the boat" entirely. Asking adolescents "What options do you have in this situation?" or "What are some different things you could try?" can prompt them to think about their available alternatives. Following such questions with a casual suggestion for further involvement (e.g., "How about jotting down the pros and cons for each idea, and letting me know what you think?") can prompt the sensible evaluation of alternatives and the selection of a new solution. Parents who are overly directive with their teens may risk alienating them, but asking questions, making casual suggestions, and asking for teens' opinions can often engage the teens more productively in problem-solving discussions. This approach demonstrates parental willingness to be helpful while at the same time respecting adolescent autonomy.

Parents often understand the benefits of helping their children learn to use problem solving, but that does not mean they can always teach problem solving effectively. Teaching problem solving takes time, and at the end of a long day it is often easier for a parent to tell the child "Just do it *this* way!" rather than attempting to elicit various alternatives. Other parents find it hard to watch their child struggle with unsuccessful solutions, and would rather "rescue" their child by solving the problem for him or her. Parents who recognize these patterns in themselves can sometimes change them, especially if given a clear rationale by their therapist. I sometimes refer back to an old adage about fishing: it is easier to catch a fish than to teach people to fish, but catching a fish feeds them for a day, while teaching them to fish feeds them for a lifetime. Problem solving is a lifetime skill; so, teaching it is well worth the effort.

FAMILY-FOCUSED PROBLEM SOLVING

When solving a problem requires the involvement of several family members and the child is old enough and cooperative enough to participate, it may make sense to do family-focused problem solving. Before starting, however, it is helpful for the therapist to understand something about family patterns relevant to problem solving and to answer the questions outlined in Table 10.1 with respect to the particular family he or she is seeing.

Family Patterns Relevant to Problem Solving

There are numerous theoretical approaches to understanding family dynamics (Combrinck-Graham, 1990), but for simplicity only patterns relevant to problem solving will be described. These patterns involve the family's overall degree of organization and flexibility, the various fam-

TABLE 10.1. Questions to Consider When Problem Solving with Families

General question	Specific issues
Is this family likely to be able to do problem solving successfully, or is another intervention needed first?	• If individual family members have psychological problems likely to affect problem solving, are they able to acknowledge and address these? • If there are patterns of family interaction likely to affect problem solving, are the adults in the family able to acknowledge and address these? • Is the degree of conflict or negative emotion in the family likely to prevent successful problem solving? • Are family members able to accept one another's different points of view to allow successful problem solving? • Is the family organized and committed enough to treatment to attend sessions consistently and to implement new solutions consistently?
Who in the family will participate in problem solving?	• Who is cognitively mature enough to participate? • Who is willing to participate? • Who is living under the same roof or struggling with the same issue? • Do there have to be different solutions for different households?
Are there factors that will limit the range of solutions considered?	• Are family members willing and able to consider solutions outside their usual family roles and family alliances? • Will limited family resources (e.g., time, money, energy) constrain the range of solutions considered? • Will cultural expectations (e.g., of the therapist, of the children) restrict the range of solutions considered?

ily members' relative power within the family, and the typical styles of family interaction.

Difficulties focusing on problem-solving steps (i.e., low organization) or generating multiple alternatives (i.e., low flexibility) have been described in the earlier section on parent-focused problem solving. Family members' relative power in the family matters because solutions proposed by more powerful members are more likely to be implemented than those proposed by less powerful members, and it is developmentally appropriate for parents to have somewhat more power than children. Relative power is not difficult to assess. For example, one can say to the family, "Please tell me about the problem that brings you here today. Anyone may start." The person who speaks first usually has the most power in the family unless he or she is being forced to speak by another, more powerful, member (e.g., through a stern look or an order to speak). The person whose recorded voice is heard on the family answering machine usually also has a high degree of power in the family. For example, when the voice is that of a young child, this may indicate that parents are indulgent or are having difficulties with setting limits. Even in families that try to appear democratic in the initial interview, members' relative power is usually obvious within a couple of sessions.

For successful problem solving, power relationships in the family should be clear to the therapist and family rather than covert, and parents should have somewhat more power than children but not be abusing that power autocratically. If a therapist notices that covert power dynamics seem to be at play in a family, it may be advisable to recommend family therapy, as exploring such dynamics usually goes beyond the scope of problem-solving techniques. Children with a high degree of power are sometimes given inappropriate adult responsibilities (e.g., involvement in decisions about family finances or responsibility in looking after a parent's emotional needs). As a result, these children may expect to be consulted on all problem-solving decisions, even those more appropriately made by their parents. On the other hand, children in families where parents are autocratic know they have no influence on family decisions, and so they are unlikely to participate in problem-solving discussions. Problem solving tends to be most effective with families where everyone can contribute ideas and everyone is listened to respectfully but where parents have the final say on important decisions. As therapists, we should encourage this style of interaction whenever possible.

Most theorists agree that family interactions are cyclical. In other words, one person's actions elicit certain reactions from another, and that person's response in turn elicits a reaction from the first person, and so on, until it is no longer clear who started the interaction. Cycles of interaction can also involve multiple family members; for example, two members may often argue until a third member intervenes. Because these habitual cycles are characteristics of the family system, no one person is blamed for them, but all members have a responsibility to change them if they are problematic.

One style of family interaction, termed "high expressed emotion," has been consistently associated with mental health problems and is also problematic when doing family-focused problem solving (Wearden, Tarrier, Barrowclough, Zastowny, & Rahill, 2000). This style is characterized by frequent interpersonal conflict and family interactions where members exacerbate one another's negative emotions. When problem solving, a family with this style might respond as follows:

THERAPIST: Let's see if we can come up with some ideas that would help Rico get to school on time. Any thoughts?

MOTHER: Well, if he wasn't texting his friends all night, maybe he could get out of bed in the morning.

RICO: Yeah, right, go blaming my friends again. If it was up to you, I'd be completely antisocial. You never let me go anywhere on weekends!

MOTHER: I never let you go anywhere? Didn't I drive you to that pool party last Saturday even though your father needed to get to the hardware store? And what thanks do I get? You never lift a finger around the house to help.

RICO: That's all you care about—your stupid house. You blame me for texting all night, but you spend the whole night cleaning!

MOTHER: Well, if you weren't such a slob, maybe I wouldn't have to! And don't you call our home stupid. You should be thankful you have a roof over your head ...

In this argumentative family, the therapist will be hard-pressed to find an opportunity to say anything, let alone guide and encourage family problem solving! One simple suggestion he or she could offer would be for both Rico and his mother to slow down and start each of their statements with "I feel ... " rather than "You do. ... " This simple strategy often reduces mutual blaming. Asking each person to paraphrase or summarize what the other person has just said is also sometimes helpful in improving communication. When people cannot follow these suggestions, however, systemic family therapy may be indicated before attempting further problem solving.

Other challenging family styles include families that only come for help when they encounter a crisis, preventing follow-up and evaluation of new solutions tried, and families that cannot implement new solutions because they challenge the family "status quo." In the latter situation, family members may verbally agree to a particular course of action but report the next week that, for one reason or another, it didn't happen. The following week, there will be another excuse as to why it didn't happen, and so on. In these families, there may be unwritten rules about what is or is not permissible, or there may be patterns of interaction among certain dyads in the family that prevent implementation of the proposed solution.

For example, family members verbally agreed to encourage a shy 13-year-old girl to take the bus more independently, but neither parent found the time to get her to the bus stop or check the bus schedule. When the therapist commented on this unfortunate lack of progress, the mother reassured, "Oh, it's not so bad. You never know who she could run into out there. Maybe we should work on something else." Further inquiry revealed that the parents had previously lived in an unsafe area where several young women had been sexually assaulted near bus stops, and they were therefore unwilling to allow their daughter to travel independently even though others were encouraging them to do so. Open discussion of these concerns and of ways of encouraging age-appropriate independence safely allowed this family to continue problem solving successfully.

Dyadic interactions that can interfere with problem solving include overly close dyads (sometimes called "enmeshment"), distant dyads, conflicted dyads, and pursuit–withdrawal patterns. In enmeshed dyads, the two family members may not be able to overtly disagree (even if they disagree covertly) or may not be able to implement solutions that require them to work separately or to not help each other. Distant dyads may not be emotionally invested enough in each other's well-being to bother working together. Conflicted dyads may not be able to work together to implement solutions, as they repeatedly clash when they attempt to do so. In pursuit–withdrawal patterns, the first person (the pursuer) may be very invested in implementing the solution and tries to get the second person (the withdrawer) to participate. The second person withdraws, however, causing the first person to intensify pursuit, prompting even more withdrawal, and so on, in a frustrating pattern that leads nowhere. All of these patterns can be challenged if identified, and some families can change them with effort and practice. If the two parties cannot change them readily, however, systemic family therapy may be indicated before engaging in family-focused problem solving.

Is Another Intervention Needed First?

Discussion of various family patterns has led us to the first general question in Table 10.1: "Is this family likely to be able to do problem solving successfully, or is another intervention needed first?" Examples of different types of interventions that may be needed first include systemic family therapy to address high expressed emotion or other problematic family interaction patterns (see above) and individual treatment for family members with significant mental health problems. Marital therapy may also be indicated if parental disagreements occur in multiple areas (i.e., not just childrearing concerns) or if either partner expresses significant marital dissatisfaction. In all cases, family members who are able to acknowledge and understand their difficulties rather than blaming one another or blaming the therapist are likely to have positive outcomes and be able to engage in problem solving later. As mentioned earlier, a certain level of family organization—allowing for consistent, focused work together and openness in the family to different points of view or to different solutions—are prerequisites for successful problem solving.

Who Will Participate?

Participants in problem-solving discussions should be cognitively mature enough to understand the problem and be able to contribute relevant ideas to the discussion. Most school-age children fit this description unless the problem is clearly of an adult nature (e.g., problems related to family finances). In fact, young children's honesty about what they observe in the family can sometimes add an interesting dimension to problem-solving discussions and result in more effective solutions. For example, a solution that required a father and son to work together elicited giggles from the family's 8-year-old daughter. "Daddy would go bananas if he had to explain all that to Jeff [his son]," she laughed. "Shut up!" scowled Jeff. The father then acknowledged his difficulty with implementing the proposed solution, and another solution was found.

It is helpful to think about the other end of the age spectrum as well. Grandparents or other relatives living under the same roof with the nuclear family being seen in therapy may have useful information to contribute and may need to be part of certain solutions. Some parents, for example, seek the approval of their own parents before implementing new childrearing strategies, especially if they live with them in the same home.

In divorced or reconstituted families, family problem-solving discussions may involve one, two, three, or four parents, depending on whether or not the biological parents' new partners are included. The decision of whom to include depends not only on the nature of the problem but also on how civil various adults act toward one another. If the relationships among the adults involved in parenting are amicable, involving them all may generate the largest number of solutions and allow for the most consistent implementation of whatever new solution is chosen. If they can barely sit in the same room together without arguing, problem solving may need to be done separately with each household. Then, the therapist needs to ensure that the children are clear about what will be done differently in each household before the families begin implementing new solutions.

Sometimes certain family members prefer not to be involved in problem-solving discussions. For example, parents may want to engage in problem-solving discussions with their teens about improving homework completion; and the teens may not be interested in participating in these discussions. In this case, the therapist has a few options. First, the therapist could try to redefine the problem in terms acceptable to the teen (or other uncooperative family member). "Reducing all the arguing at homework time," for example, may be a more acceptable goal for a teen than increasing homework completion. Sometimes this approach allows for a fruitful problem-solving discussion, but it is also possible that the teen may either persist in not participating or contribute only ideas that involve changing his or her parents' behavior. In the latter situation, the therapist could explain that "everyone has to help a little" if things are to change, to encourage more balanced solutions. If the teen continues to resist participating, it is usually advisable to work primarily with the parents. Parents may be discouraged by their teen's refusal to participate; so, the therapist may need to emphasize the parents' ability to *model* appropriate behavior and the teen's ability to learn from the consequences of his or her own behavior. For example, parents could model finishing chores before watching television. They could also indicate that they will not nag the teen about homework but will do a weekly check-in with his or her teachers. If the teachers indicate no problems, the parents will praise the teen for improvement, and the frequency of their check-ins will be reduced. If problems are reported, the parents will withdraw a privilege and increase the frequency of check-ins.

Regardless of the solution chosen, reducing emotional reactions to their children's negative behavior is a universally helpful parenting strategy. Some parents can reduce these reactions in response to some education by the therapist about the consequences of negative emotional reactions. In brief, negative emotional reactions by parents increase attention to the child or teen's bad behavior. Because children value attention negative emotional reactions inadvertently reinforce bad behavior and thus increase the behavior's frequency. Conversely, deliberately ignoring bad behavior decreases attention, and therefore often decreases the frequency of the behavior. Of course, severe misbehavior that could harm others or is illegal cannot be ignored and must be addressed with appropriate consequences. Deliberate ignoring is a helpful strategy for decreasing minor misbehaviors, however, and many parents can master it with practice. Parents who are unable to curtail negative emotional reactions to their children's behavior despite repeated efforts may need help discovering the reasons for these reactions, either through personal psychotherapy or family therapy.

What Types of Solutions Are "Off Limits"?

The types of solutions families are willing to consider can be constrained by several factors. These include family dynamics (see above), family resources, and cultural expectations.

Solutions that require more time, money, or energy than family members possess are unlikely to work. Unfortunately, families are not always forthcoming with information about these limitations. Many people, for example, will nod pleasantly when someone suggests implementing a particular solution, not implement it because of resource constraints, and then make vague excuses about why nothing was done or simply not come back to sessions. For example, one young boy was problem solving with his peers in woodworking class about how to build a bird house together. The group agreed that each member would bring one tool or one of the materials for the next class. The boy agreed to bring some nails, but when he asked for money to go to the hardware store his father replied, "After I get paid next week." Ashamed, the boy skipped the next class rather than facing his peers. Therapists are wise to ask about families' financial circumstances before suggesting new solutions and to supply necessary materials (e.g., tokens for public transit to get to sessions and stationery for any paperwork between sessions) if the family's poverty is a consideration.

Lack of time or lack of energy for implementation can be a realistic constraint too, especially in single-parent families with several children or in families where one or more members are ill or have special needs. For example, a depressed single parent raising one autistic child and a second child with behavior problems is unlikely to have much energy to implement new solutions to address the second child's behaviors. Providing temporary care for the autistic child to allow for parental respite (and perhaps some added time to bond with the second child) is more likely to be helpful than blaming this parent for failing to implement new solutions. Respite care for developmentally disabled children is available in many jurisdictions, but parents may need a physician's or the therapist's referral to access these services.

Assumptions based on cultural background may also limit the range of solutions some families are willing to consider or implement. Such assumptions may not be obvious, especially if family members speak fluent English, but these assumptions can undermine problem solving if not explicitly discussed. In talking to families, therapists should be alert for body language or facial expressions suggesting discomfort with certain ideas or solutions. Then they can ask, "Are you comfortable with that idea?", "What bothers you about that idea?", or "Would this be an acceptable solution in your culture or not?" to elicit culturally relevant information. With such information, solutions can often be found that are both culturally sensitive and effective.

If no solution appears acceptable to the family, one could consider involving an elder or professional from that culture (if available) to interpret what is culturally normative in a given situation. Thus, I have sometimes involved clergy from particular religious groups to clarify the acceptable options for certain situations. A child who had panic attacks whenever she went to mass, for example, revealed that statues of Jesus being crucified were giving her nightmares, but her family feared for her soul if she did not attend religious services. A discussion with the family's priest revealed that it was acceptable for her to avoid mass or sit away from the frightening statues until she had a chance to discuss and deal with her fears.

Culturally based assumptions can pertain to the role of the therapist, the role of the parents, and the role of the children. For example, in some cultures doctors or healers are revered and expected to give sage advice rather than (as in problem solving) eliciting ideas from those who seek their help. Families from these cultures may look to the therapist to tell them what to do rather than making decisions themselves using problem solving. In some cultures, parents have very clearly defined gender roles. For example, childrearing may be seen as the mother's responsibility, and so solutions that involve the father may be frowned upon. Some cultures emphasize children's duty to give their parents respect, loyalty, and support as they age rather than emphasizing (as North American culture typically does) parents' duty to provide their children with every reasonable opportunity to realize their potential. For families from these cultures, implementing a solution suggested by a child rather than a parent may seem foreign or inappropriate.

Even within North America, however, there are subcultures that will only consider certain types of solutions. For example, some families regularly visit practitioners of complementary medical approaches such as homeopathy or naturopathy. These families may insist that whatever solution is implemented must be "natural" or "holistic," and they tend to shy away from conventional medical approaches. As with any cultural difference (see above), therapists should be alert for body language or facial expressions suggesting discomfort with certain ideas or solutions, explore reasons for the discomfort, and seek solutions that are both culturally sensitive and effective. Only solutions that are clearly harmful to the child should not be considered. Generally, however, the best solutions are ones that families are eager to implement, and therefore they must be consistent with families' values.

Despite the challenges involved, problem solving with families can be very rewarding. As in group problem solving, "Many heads are better than one"—so many more creative solutions are possible when working with families than when working with individuals. In addition, the value family members place on their relationships with one another often makes families highly motivated to participate in problem solving. Furthermore, establishing family problem solving as a means of addressing difficulties can have a huge impact on children's development. Many children are raised in environments where solutions are either imposed (e.g., "Do it because I said so") or argued about but rarely implemented. Learning that difficulties can be overcome in ways that include everyone's input and that actually work is a wonderful lesson that children learn when their families begin to use problem solving successfully.

Chapter 11

Troubleshooting

Even the most skilled therapists occasionally encounter unexpected obstacles in their work. This chapter describes some common obstacles one might encounter when using problem solving with children and families and how to address these issues. Some obstacles are specific to problem solving, while others occur in many types of psychotherapy. Obstacles that are specific to problem solving relate to the pragmatic nature of this therapeutic technique, the emotional meaning of the problem in the client's life, inconsistency or other chronic implementation difficulties, or unrealistic client expectations. Obstacles that can occur in any form of psychotherapy relate to unhelpful therapist and client attitudes and to the therapeutic relationship.

THERAPEUTIC OBSTACLES
SPECIFIC TO PROBLEM SOLVING

The Pragmatic Nature of Problem Solving

When we employ problem-solving as a therapeutic technique, we assume that the client is presenting a problem because he or she wants help in finding a practical solution for it. This assumption is not always correct. Consider this conversation between Isabelle, age 14, and her father.

ISABELLE: I'd like to go to the team lunch, but I don't think I can get there. It's at a restaurant across town, and you and Mom will both be at work today at lunchtime.

FATHER: Well, why don't you call one of your older friends and see if you can get a ride? We could also look at the bus schedule and see if there's a bus that runs across town at that time, ... and Milly [a retired next-door neighbor] might be able to drive you.

ISABELLE: Oh, Dad, you just don't get it!

Isabelle's father is puzzled and hurt by her reaction, but it's not an unusual one. If he had allowed Isabelle to talk more about the lunch before offering solutions, Isabelle's father would have learned that she was ambivalent about going because she was planning to use the day to prepare for an important examination. Thus, although Isabelle appeared to present her father a problem to be solved, she was really hoping that he would listen empathically to her concerns. With his support and empathy, she could then make up her mind more easily about what to do.

Some authors (most famously John Gray in *Men Are from Mars, Women Are from Venus* [1992]) suggest that Isabelle's style of communication, which is more common in females than males, plays a role in interpersonal conflicts between men and women. Regardless of age or gender, however, people sometimes prefer a good listener to a problem solver. An astute therapist should consider this possibility when the client demonstrates an unexpected negative reaction to problem solving.

The Problem Serves an Emotional Purpose

Another assumption therapists often naturally make is that the client wants to eliminate the problem. Sometimes, however, the problem serves a useful emotional purpose in the life of the child or the lives of other family members. A child who appears to be anxious about going to school, for example, may feel needed at home to offer support to a depressed parent. Problem solving strictly focused on returning to school is unlikely to succeed under these circumstances. Alternatively, a child whose parents have a conflicted relationship may misbehave repeatedly at school, resulting in frequent parent–teacher conferences. Problem solving that eliminates the misbehavior might reduce the parents' need to work together, destabilizing the parental relationship. In this case, the "problem" of child misbehavior may be keeping the family together!

Even if the child only has a vague awareness of these family dynamics, he or she is likely to continue to be motivated to behave poorly.

Consider the dilemma that Robbie, an 8-year-old boy, encountered. Robbie's mother had a very stressful job, and one strategy that came up in a session was for Robbie to learn to make his own school lunches so that his mother would no longer be burdened with this task. He appeared to be cooperating with a problem-solving approach to this issue, but then he suddenly tearfully burst out, "If I can't even be with my mom to make lunch, I'll never see her during the week!" Further discussion revealed that there was some truth to this exclamation: his mother rarely spent time with Robbie except on the weekends. Thus, learning to make lunch independently would deprive the boy of a brief but precious opportunity to interact with his mother. In this case, the therapist wisely chose to focus on increasing Robbie's ability to perform other independent behaviors that did not interfere with mother–son time. She also talked to Robbie's mother about adjusting her work schedule to allow more time to look after herself and her family.

Clues that suggest that a problem serves an emotional purpose include:

- An unexpected negative reaction by the child or another family member to a problem-solving attempt.
- Repeated lack of success in implementing various solutions to a given problem.
- The emergence of a different but similar problem as soon as one problem is solved (e.g., lack of homework completion is replaced by not completing chores; disruptive behavior at school is replaced by disruptive behavior at friends' houses; conflict with teachers is replaced by conflict with peers).
- Parents who always report a new problem in a particular child as soon as one has been solved.

The final point merits further exploration, as such a situation can occur for several reasons. Sometimes parents have difficulty liking their child even when his or her behavior improves, indicated by their constantly finding new faults with the child. This can occur when there is a temperamental mismatch between parent and child (for example, an athletically gifted child with poor grades in a highly intellectual family; a boy who is a talented dancer in a family that considers dance effeminate) or when the child is being made a scapegoat for other family problems. Sometimes the parents like their child but are very anxious about him or her (perhaps because the child has a serious medical condition, or possibly because of an anxiety disorder in the parent). An anxious parent will often report multiple problems about a child even when most of these are not interfering significantly with the child's life. Some parents also have a strong need to remain involved in their children's lives to a greater degree than is developmentally appropriate and may not be consciously aware of this need. For example, one clever 12-year-old whose mother asked multiple questions about various aspects of school that might be problematic eventually piped up, "Oh, Mom! Are you looking for another problem so you can intervene again?" Fortunately, his mother responded with a good-natured laugh, as she recognized this pattern of behavior in herself. Thus, there can be many reasons for the "multiproblem child," and they are well worth clarifying.

Repeated Difficulties with Implementation

Many difficulties with implementation were already discussed in Chapter 6. Here are a few more to consider in relation to two typical comments by children or parents.

1. "I/We didn't get to it this week" (repeated for 3 consecutive weeks). Possibilities include:
   - The client lacks a skill needed to implement the solution.
   - The client verbally agreed to the solution but is not comfortable with it (e.g., an adolescent who fears the new solution will cause embarrassment).
   - The client needs help from others to implement the solution but is uncomfortable asking for it.
   - Implementing the new solution does not fit in with child's or family's lifestyle (e.g., evidenced by a seeming lack of time to devote to the new solution even when considerable efforts have been made to fit it in).
   - Other people are interfering with implementing the new solution (e.g., meddling relatives, or teachers who are not convinced the solution will work).
   - The the problem serves an emotional purpose (see above).
2. "I/We tried but it's not working/there's no difference." Possibilities include:
   - Implementation is inconsistent.
   - Logistical problems or negative emotions are interfering with successful implementation.

- Change has occurred, but the client(s) is not aware of it.
- Client(s)' expectations of change are unrealistic.

Inconsistency

Inconsistency can occur between people and across time. Find out exactly where and when the child and family attempted to implement the solution, what exactly was done, and who participated. For example, a family of a teen who spent hours on social networking sites at the expense of his homework agreed to use "Facebook time" as a reward for finishing school work. Initially, his father monitored the young man's computer access, and the solution appeared to be working. However, after a few days his father stopped doing so, and things changed. Since some school work required computer access and neither parent was monitoring that access, the boy claimed to be doing homework while actually connecting with his friends online. Clearly, consistent monitoring needed to be part of this solution, or else it was unlikely to succeed.

Inconsistency can also occur between parents or between home and school. For example, if parents agree to a bedtime routine that facilitates independent sleep for a child, it is important that both parents follow exactly the same routine. If one parent remains with the child for 10 minutes and then leaves the room but the other does not leave until the child falls asleep, the child's ability to fall sleep independently is unlikely to improve. Home and school differences often occur when the new solution is described in vague terms. For example, a school teacher and two parents agreed that a child should be rewarded for "independent work." The parents did a sample question for the child and then rewarded each subsequent question the child answered without assistance. The school teacher, on the other hand, expected the child to begin the questions independently (i.e., no sample question provided) and wondered why so little progress was evident. To reiterate: clarify precisely what was done where, when, and by whom to identify hidden inconsistencies. Then, use a problem-solving approach to increase consistency.

Logistical Problems

Logistical problems are usually obvious. For example, suppose a child is working on taking the bus back and forth to school, but the bus schedule does not allow him or her to attend after-school soccer practice. If soccer is the child's favorite sport, the child may not be motivated to take the bus at the end of the school day.

Negative Emotions

Negative emotions, on the other hand, are not always obvious because people are sometimes reluctant to acknowledge them. Parents who argue with their children in an attempt to change their children's behavior, for example, may not be proud of these arguments, especially since they are usually impossible to win. Arguing, however, is one of the most common factors that can undermine successful implementation. When parents argue with their children, they pay attention to them. Unfortunately, children find extra parental attention rewarding even if it is negative. For this reason, arguments often increase the very behavior the parent is trying to decrease. If a therapist suspects this difficulty, it may be helpful to normalize arguing (e.g., "All families disagree sometimes, and many end up arguing over their disagreements. Does that happen at your house?"). Once the arguing is acknowledged, it can be identified as something that interferes with implementation, and alternatives to arguing can be discussed.

Lack of Awareness of Change

Lack of awareness of change can sometimes result in discouraging reports that "nothing is getting any better." It is human nature to block out the worst aspects of a situation; so, small improvements are sometimes discounted. Refer back to Chapter 3, where baseline measures were discussed. If a baseline of a problem's severity has been done, it is relatively easy to refer back to it and see if there has been any progress. If no baseline has been done previously, do one at the time of the discouraging report, and encourage consistent implementation for a couple of weeks. Then redo the measure to get an accurate evaluation of change. If there has been slight progress, encourage perseverance with the solution used. If there has been no progress, help the client move on to a different solution, using the measure of the problem's severity at that time as the new baseline.

Unrealistic Expectations

Sometimes, despite careful preparation by the therapist, children and families pursue problem solving with unrealistic expectations of change. Here are some comments that suggest that client expectations need to be adjusted, along with some helpful responses to them:

- *Parent:* "I don't want to change anything. I just want her to be happy and well behaved."

- *Response:* Unhappy, badly behaving children are unlikely to become happy and well behaved simply because a parent wishes for this outcome or because a therapist performs some sort of magic trick. Children change in response to changes in their environment and sometimes because of their own willingness to try something new. As adults, it is up to us to create environments for and relationships with our children that foster positive change. Problem solving is one approach that can be used to do this. Some child behaviors may improve with maturation, but there is no guarantee this will occur.

- *Adolescent:* "I'm not going to do anything different. Just get my parents off my back!"

- *Response:* "I wish I could get your parents off your back, but they're unlikely to budge right now. Do you know why? I think they're worried about you, and as long as they're worried they will keep checking up on you. Maybe there's a way to reassure them so they can stop monitoring your every move. Would it be worth figuring that out? Let's see what we can come up with."

- *Parent:* "Just make her feel better first, then she can try it" or "His self-esteem is too low to try that right now."

- *Response:* Usually, children need to do better before they feel better. An exception to this rule occurs when the child or teen has a serious mental illness (e.g., a psychotic illness or clinical depression) that may need treatment before the child's functioning can improve. If this is not the case, however, children usually feel better about themselves as a result of better behavior. Doing well makes us all feel more competent and more confident than doing poorly. Often it also results in positive feedback from others, which makes us feel even better. Therefore, encouraging children to try new solutions is usually more helpful than waiting for their feelings or self-esteem to improve.

- *Parent:* "Find the root cause of the problem first; then we can solve it."

- *Response:* Problem solving focuses on the here and now, not remote causes from the distant past. Sometimes the past is relevant, but it is surprising how many people can find and implement successful solutions to their problems despite an unfortunate past history. If there are emotional reasons for maintaining a problem (see above), these should be addressed. However, if it is clear that the problem is one that you want to solve, there is no reason to delay doing so.

- *Child:* "I've come up with some good ideas. Now, tell me the right answer!"

- *Response:* The answer that is best will be different for each person. Some people might do best with *this* idea ... some people might do better with *that* idea. We have to try them out to see which one works best for you.

- *Parent:* "I know we've solved the problem, but she's still not enthusiastic about it."

- *Response:* As adults, we can help children change their behavior, but they are not always going to like it. Change is hard for anyone, children included. Expecting a child to embrace it enthusiastically is simply too much to ask.

THERAPEUTIC OBSTACLES ENCOUNTERED IN MANY TYPES OF PSYCHOTHERAPY

Some therapeutic obstacles are not unique to problem solving. These include both unhelpful therapist and client attitudes toward therapy and problems in the therapist–client relationship.

Unhelpful Therapist Attitudes toward Therapy

Some therapists have misgivings about using problem solving in their work. There are different reasons for these misgivings. If you are uncomfortable using problem solving in your therapeutic work, see if one of the following four descriptions rings true:

1. A therapist may have a strong need to give advice to clients. After all, it feels good to provide helpful suggestions to clients, and clients are often grateful for them. When using problem solving, however, it is important to curtail this tendency in order to allow the client to learn from experience what is most helpful for his or her difficulties. Watching clients struggle with imperfect solutions can be hard, and it is tempting to jump in and tell them what to do. However, it is useful to remember that clients must not only solve their current problems but also develop the skills to solve future problems. Otherwise, they remain dependent on you, the therapist, whenever a new problem arises. Following the prob-

lem-solving steps without giving definitive advice helps people develop those skills, allowing them to find solutions that work for them with increasingly greater independence.

2. A therapist may have been taught (e.g., when training in psychodynamic psychotherapy) to be nondirective in order to allow the client's thoughts and feelings to emerge. For this therapist, problem solving may seem too structured and directive for comfort. Its emphasis on practical solutions rather than the client's inner world may also make it seem somewhat superficial. For this therapist, it is useful to remember that practical successes can have a profoundly positive effect on the client's thoughts and feelings even if those thoughts and feelings are not explored in detail.

3. A therapist may consider problem solving simplistic or mundane as compared to other therapeutic techniques. For example, there is a certain pride he or she may experience when making brilliant interpretations in psychodynamic psychotherapy or when identifying the client's key cognitive distortions in CBT. This pride is rarely experienced when using problem solving. In problem solving, we must take pride in our clients' successes rather than our own. Therefore, deliberately focusing on the client's success is often helpful for this therapist.

4. A therapist may lack confidence in his or her ability to help the client solve problems. Inexperienced therapists or therapists who struggle in their personal lives with similar problems to those of their clients sometimes feel this way. It is sometimes helpful for these clinicians to remember that it is not the therapist's job to always be an expert problem solver. It is all right to learn some aspects of problem solving together with our clients.

Unhelpful Client Attitudes toward Therapy

Unhelpful client attitudes toward problem solving often mirror those of their therapists, which is important to consider if a client appears unhappy.

Another possibility is that the client is not fully engaged in problem solving because he or she is unsure how it can be helpful. If you suspect this to be the case, review with the client the relationship between the problem that is currently the focus of therapy and other problems that he or she may encounter. The goal of problem solving is not just to solve a single problem, which may seem trivial to the client, but to develop a set of skills for solving all kinds of problems that may occur in the client's life. Other reasons for lack of engagement or lack of motivation have already been discussed in Chapter 2 and should also be reviewed.

Finally, it is possible that the client is fully engaged in problem solving but progress is being undermined by a secret difficulty that he or she has not disclosed to the therapist. Untreated substance abuse, for example, can undermine even the best problem-solving efforts in adolescents and adults. Similarly, if there are parental plans for family separation but these have not been shared with the child or with the therapist, these can undermine problem solving in children. For example, a child may be problem solving a particular difficulty with peers at school while not realizing that his or her school placement is about to change as a result of his or her parents' divorce.

Problems in the Therapist–Client Relationship

The work of psychotherapy can only proceed if there is a close but respectful relationship between therapist and client. Trust and effective communication are essential to this relationship but are not always easy to establish. To begin, let us consider the challenges of establishing trust.

Clients and therapists begin their work together as strangers, but clients are expected to eventually entrust even the most intimate details of their lives to their therapists. It is important that therapists not abuse that trust and that they use the information they learn to benefit the client. Some children, adolescents, and families begin therapy after negative past experiences with other therapists or with other important people in their lives who they felt took advantage of or betrayed them. These experiences may make it difficult for them to trust you. If so, be open with them about how hard it can be to trust someone after feeling betrayed, and patiently persevere even if the client's involvement in therapy initially seems limited or superficial.

Occasionally, in rare cases, it is not possible to establish a trusting therapeutic relationship. Past hurts are too fresh or too severe for the client to work with any therapist. Children who have been recently abused or repeatedly abused in the past sometimes fall into this category. They may need to be in a stable, caring home environment for months or even years before they can trust an adult sufficiently to engage in psychotherapy.

Although trust is fundamental to a therapeutic relationship, other aspects are important too (see Green, 2010, for a more detailed review). The client and therapist need to work together productively, and that productive work requires good communication. Turn taking, for example, can be difficult if the client is either overly talkative or very withdrawn. Children with ADHD often talk a great deal, but much of what they say may be off topic. They benefit from regular redirection by the therapist and sometimes from taking breaks during sessions to reduce the need for sustained attention. Withdrawn children, on the other hand, may need to be drawn out by the therapist. Asking specific rather than open-ended questions may reduce awkward silences. Praise and encouragement for every small contribution the child makes to the session is also helpful. Some therapists also use drawing or play materials to help the child warm up to talking in the session.

Once a pattern of communication between the therapist and client is established, the therapist must be alert to signs of miscommunication. Some youngsters tell their therapists when they feel misunderstood, but rolling eyes, an apathetic posture, or a sullen expression may also suggest this has occurred. Summarize what you think the child or adolescent has said, and ask for confirmation that this is correct. Usually this approach clarifies what has gone wrong. If not, comment on the body language that suggests miscommunication, or hazard a guess as to what is happening. For example, say, "You look kind of annoyed today. I wonder if I missed something you were trying to say."

A negative client reaction is also possible when communication has been clear but he or she interprets it in a negative way because it reminds him or her of negative past experiences outside of therapy. Termed "transference" by psychodynamic psychotherapists, this phenomenon can occur in all forms of psychotherapy. Consider the case of Brittany, a young teen trying to develop problem-solving skills to cope better with high school.

> BRITTANY: I got a bad mark on my assignment because I missed the due date. Stupid teacher! She told everyone the due date the day I was at the track meet.
>
> KM: Sorry to hear that, Brittany. What could you do to keep on top of due dates from now on?
>
> BRITTANY: Nothing! The teacher's just picking on people on the track team.
>
> KM: Could you ask a friend for the notes from class when you go to a meet?
>
> BRITTANY: Oh, sure, now it's my job to fix it! (*Continues in a nasal, pedantic voice.*) You're in grade 9 now, Brittany. It's *your* responsibility.

KM: Oops! Did I just react like your mom? Sorry about that. Would you like to move on to a different issue or continue with this one?

BRITTANY: Well, I don't like getting bad grades, so I guess we should keep going, but I still think the teacher should do more.

KM: OK. Let's see if we can come up with an idea that gets the teacher more involved.

Brittany eventually decided to tell her teacher about upcoming track meets so she could get the work assignments that would be covered in class in advance. Her strategy was successful and her grades improved.

In this case, the pedantic tone of voice Brittany used to mimic her mother made the transference reaction obvious. By labeling it and responding differently than her mother typically did (i.e., giving her a choice instead of telling her what to do), I was able to defuse the tension in the conversation and get Brittany to work with me again. Transference reactions can be more subtle, though, so it is worth being alert to this possibility whenever you encounter an unexpected negative client reaction.

Keep in mind also that as therapists we too are subject to emotional reactions that stem from the past. The formal term for this is "countertransference." Simply put, some clients seem to "push our buttons" even when they say things that are objectively quite innocuous. For example, some therapists have a difficult time with clients who repeatedly present themselves as victims of circumstance, while others have a harder time with those who claim to be self-sufficient masters of their own destiny, never needing anyone's help. The difference is probably attributable to past experiences the therapist has had in close relationships outside of work (e.g., relationships with parents, siblings, or intimate partners). By identifying these personal biases, we can often avoid overreacting to our clients and become more helpful to them.

ADDITIONAL RESPONSES
TO THERAPEUTIC OBSTACLES

By identifying and addressing the therapeutic obstacles discussed above, it is often possible to continue successful problem solving with the client. Sometimes, however, it is either not possible to identify the source of the difficulty or not possible to resolve the difficulty despite some understanding of its source. In this case, there are several options.

If the source of the difficulty is clear and the difficulty is clearly not amenable to problem solving, one can move on to another therapeutic technique. For example, if the client has very negative attitudes toward problem solving and it is not possible to change these, it may be advisable to try a different approach. Similarly, if a family has very strict rules that prevent the exploration of a variety of solutions, it may not be possible to continue with problem solving. Given the amount of work clients and therapists often invest in the therapeutic relationship (see above), it is usually preferable to change the technique rather than change to a new therapist.

If the source of the difficulty is either not clear or it seems clear but repeated attempts to address it have failed, it may be worth arranging a consultation with a colleague. Consultations can be obtained informally, especially if one works in a group practice or mental health organization. An informal conversation with a colleague is often easier and quicker to arrange than a formal referral to another mental health professional. It is important, however, that the informal nature of the interaction not compromise client confidentiality. Thus, such a conversation should occur in the office of either the consultant or the consultee, not in the hallway or elevator where it might be overheard by others. It should also be clear who is retaining primary responsibility for the case so that the client knows who to turn to if there are further difficulties.

Whether a consultation is sought formally or informally, it is important to pose clear questions to one's consultant and to indicate clearly the desired outcome of the consultation. Thus, it is generally not helpful to send a consultation request that states simply "Child is anxious. Please assess." Instead, indicate as clearly as possible the nature of the therapeutic impasse, including relevant background information, and what you hope the consultant can do to help. For example, a formal consultation request could read:

> "This 11-year-old boy is often anxious in response to peer teasing. We have used a problem-solving approach to help him better manage the teasing, and we involved the parents and school officials to ensure better supervision of peer interactions. Teasing has decreased, his social skills have improved, and he has several friends, but he continues to be anxious about peer situations. Please assess the reasons for his continued anxiety, and advise regarding further therapeutic interventions I could provide. Previous reports and assessments are attached."

In this case, relevant background information has been provided, the question to be answered is clear (i.e., "Why is this boy still anxious about peer situations?"), and the desired outcome is also clear (i.e., "I would like to provide this boy with more helpful therapeutic interventions"). Possible outcomes or goals of a consultation one might hope for include:

- Obtaining advice on how to optimize treatment because of lack of progress in therapy (as in the case above).
- Obtaining advice on how to optimize treatment because of difficulties in the therapeutic relationship.
- Obtaining a second opinion for the client because he or she is dissatisfied with progress or with the therapeutic relationship.
- Determining whether one should continue working with a particular client or, instead, consider referral to another professional.
- Sharing care with the consultant (i.e., the consultant provides additional intervention that complements your own).

Some people also refer clients to consultants with the hope that the consultant will take the case off their hands, and they sometimes even tell the client this might occur. This practice, however, does not constitute a legitimate use of the term "consultation." Trying to get rid of disagreeable clients by sending them to consultants is dishonest and unfair to both the client and the consultant. If the consultant has therapeutic expertise that you lack, acknowledge this fact, and suggest sharing the client's care. Most consultants appreciate this approach and will indicate quickly whether or not they have the time or ability to work with the client using a shared care model.

Most of the time, consultations provide additional perspective on a case and one or more recommendations on how to proceed. Occasionally, they conclude that further work with a particular client is unlikely to be fruitful and suggest either stopping therapy or referring the client to another professional. If this occurs, it is important not to assume that therapy has been a waste of time. Many children and teens spend a few months seeing a psychotherapist with limited progress and then stop. Nevertheless, they may remember their therapist as a benevolent, sincere adult who was as helpful as he or she was able to be. This memory may allow them to reenter another therapeutic relationship in the future, when it may have a better chance of succeeding.

Thus, sincere therapeutic efforts focused on the best interests of the young person are never wasted. Even though we cannot help all of the people all of the time, we can still treat each person as a unique individual with unique gifts, worthy of our interest and respect. I have often thought that the human race is like a jigsaw puzzle: interconnected and interdependent in ways we can hardly imagine. If so, we are truly privileged as therapists, for we can never be sure what "piece" is sitting before us and what he or she is destined to become and to do. May we make the most of this privilege.

References

Adams, J., & Adams, M. (1996). The association among negative life events, perceived problem solving alternatives, depression, and suicidal ideation in adolescent psychiatric patients. *Journal of Child Psychology and Psychiatry, 37*(6), 715–720.

Arie, M., Apter, A., Orbach, I., Yefet, Y., & Zalzman, G. (2008). Autobiographical memory, interpersonal problem solving, and suicidal behavior in adolescent inpatients. *Comprehensive Psychiatry, 49*(1), 22–29.

Barkley, R. A., Edwards, G., Laneri, M., Fletcher, K., & Metevia, L. (2001). The efficacy of problem-solving communication training alone, behavior management training alone, and their combination for parent–adolescent conflict in teenagers with ADHD and ODD. *Journal of Consulting and Clinical Psychology, 69*(6), 926–941.

Barrett, P. M., Dadds, M. R., & Rapee, R. M. (1996). Family treatment of childhood anxiety: A controlled trial. *Journal of Consulting and Clinical Psychology, 64,* 333–342.

Barrett, P. M., Rapee, R. M., Dadds, M. M., & Ryan, S. M. (1996) Family enhancement of cognitive style in anxious and aggressive children. *Journal of Abnormal Child Psychology, 24,* 187–203.

Bell, A. C., & D'Zurilla, T. J. (2009). Problem-solving therapy for depression: A meta-analysis. *Clinical Psychology Review, 29*(4), 348–353.

Berman, A., Jobes, D. A., & Silverman, M. M. (2005). *Adolescent suicide: Assessment and intervention* (2nd ed.). Washington, DC: American Psychological Association.

Bowers, M., & Pipes, R. B. (2000). Influence of consultation on ethical decision making: An analogue study. *Ethics and Behavior, 10,* 65–79.

Brody, A. E. (2009). Motivational interviewing in a depressed adolescent. *Journal of Clinical Psychology, 6*(11), 1168–1179.

Brooks, R., & Goldstein, S. (2001). *Raising resilient children*. New York: McGraw-Hill.

Burns, D. D. (1999). *Feeling good: The new mood therapy* (rev. ed.). New York: Avon Books.

Carris, M. J., Sheeber, L., & Howe, S. (1998). Family rigidity, adolescent problem-solving deficits, and suicidal ideation: A mediational model. *Journal of Adolescence, 21*(4), 459–472.

Cobb, C. L. (1996). Adolescent–parent attachments and family problem-solving styles. *Family Process, 35*(1), 57–82.

Combrinck-Graham, L. (1990). Developments in family systems theory and research. *Journal of the American Academy of Child and Adolescent Psychiatry, 29*, 501–512.

Davila, J., Hammen, C., Burge, D., Paley, B., & Daley, S. E. (1995). Poor interpersonal problem solving as a mechanism of stress generation in depression among adolescent women. *Journal of Abnormal Psychology, 104*(4), 592–600.

Dornburg, C. C., Stevens, S. M., Hendrickson, S. M., & Davidson, G. S. (2009). Improving extreme-scale problem-solving: Assessing electronic brainstorming effectiveness in an industrial setting. *Human Factors, 51*(4), 519–527.

Fagot, B. I., & Gauvain, M. (1997). Mother–child problem solving: Continuity through the early childhood years. *Developmental Psychology, 33*(3), 480–488.

Frank, A., Green, V., & McNeil, D. W. (1993). Adolescent substance users: Problem-solving abilities. *Journal of Substance Abuse, 5*(1), 85–92.

Fredelius, G., Sandell, R., & Lindqvist, C. (2002). Who should receive psychotherapy?: Analysis of decision makers' think-aloud protocols. *Qualitative Health Research, 12*, 640–654.

Goffin, S., & Tull, C. (1985). Problem solving: Encouraging active learning. *Psychology of Young Children, 40*, 28–32.

Gray, J. (1992). *Men are from Mars, women are from Venus*. New York: HarperCollins.

Green, J. (2010). *Creating the therapeutic relationship in counseling and psychotherapy*. New York: Learning Matters.

Greene, R. W. (2010). *The explosive child: A new approach for understanding and parenting easily frustrated, chronically inflexible children* (rev. & updated). New York: HarperCollins.

Greene, R. W., Ablon, J. S., Hassuk, B., Regan, K. M., & Martin, A. (2006). Innovations: Child and adolescent psychiatry: Use of collaborative problem solving to reduce seclusion and restraint in child and adolescent inpatient units. *Psychiatric Services, 57*(5), 610–612.

Greene, R. W., & Duncan, D. (2010, September). *Coerce or collaborate: Is there an alternative to behaviour therapy for ADHD and its comorbidities?* Symposium at the Canadian Academy of Child and Adolescent Psychiatry 30th Annual Conference, Toronto.

Greening, L. (1997). Adolescent stealers' and non-stealers' social problem-solving skills. *Adolescence, 32*(125), 51–55.

Hains, A. A., & Hains, A. H. (1987). The effects of a cognitive strategy intervention on the problem-solving abilities of delinquent youths. *Journal of Adolescence, 10*(4), 399–413.

Hanna, K. J., Ewart, C. K., & Kwiterovich, P. O. (1990). Child problem solving competence, behavioral adjustment and adherence to lipid-lowering diet. *Patient Education and Counseling, 16*(2), 119–131.

Hops, H., Tildesley, E., Lichtenstein, E., Ary, D., & Sherman, L. (1990). Parent-adolescent problem-solving interactions and drug use. *American Journal of Drug and Alcohol Abuse, 16*(3–4), 239–258.

Jaffee, W. B., & D'Zurilla, T. J. (2009). Personality, problem solving, and adolescent substance use. *Behavior Therapy, 40*(1), 93–101.

Jensen, P. S., Hinshaw, S. P., Swanson, J. M., Greenhill, L. L., Conners, C. K., Arnold, L. E., et al. (2001). Findings from the NIMH Multimodal Treatment Study of ADHD (MTA): Implications and applications for primary care providers. *Journal of Developmental and Behavioral Pediatrics, 22*(1), 60–73.

Kable, J. W., & Glimcher, P. W. (2010). An "as soon as possible" effect in human intertemporal decision making: Behavioral evidence and neural mechanisms. *Journal of Neurophysiology, 103*, 2513–2531.

Kazdin, A. E., Esveldt-Dawson, K., French, N. H., & Unis, A. S. (1987a). Problem-solving skills training and relationship therapy in the treatment of antisocial child behavior. *Journal of Consulting and Clinical Psychology, 55*(1), 76–85.

Kazdin, A. E., Esveldt-Dawson, K., French, N. H., & Unis, A. S. (1987b). Effects of parent management training and problem-solving skills combined in the treatment of antisocial child behavior. *Journal of the American Academy of Child and Adolescent Psychiatry, 26*(3), 416–424.

Kendall, P. C. (1992). *Stop and think workbook* (2nd ed.). Philadelphia: Workbook.

Kendall, P. C. (2006). *Coping cat workbook* (2nd ed.). Philadelphia: Workbook.

Kendall, P. C., & Bartel, N. R. (1990). *Teaching problem solving to students with learning and behavior problems*. Ardmore, PA: Workbook.

Kendall, P. C., Choudhury, M. A., Hudson, J., & Webb, A. (2002). *The C.A.T. project manual for the cognitive behavioral treatment of anxious adolescents (therapist manual)*. Philadelphia: Workbook.

Layne, A. E., Bernstein, G. A., Egan, E. A., & Kushner, M. G. (2003). Predictors of treatment response in anxious–depressed adolescents with school refusal. *Journal of the American Academy of Child and Adolescent Psychiatry, 42*, 319–326.

Lin, C. F., & Wang, H. F. (2008). A decision-making process model of young online shoppers. *Cyberpsychology and Behavior, 11*, 759–761.

Lochman, J. E., Wayland, K. K., & White, K. J. (1993). Social goals: Relationship to adolescent adjustment and to social problem-solving. *Journal of Abnormal Child Psychology, 21*(2), 135–151.

Luhmann, C. C. (2009). Temporal decision-making: Insights from cognitive neuroscience. *Frontiers in Behavioral Neuroscience, 3*, 39.

Manassis, K. (2005). Empirical data regarding the role of the family in treatment. In R. Rapee & J. Hudson (Eds.), *Current thinking on psychopathology and the family* (pp. 287–304). New York: Elsevier.

Manassis, K. (2007). *Keys to parenting your anxious child* (2nd ed.). Hauppauge, NY: Barron's.

Manassis, K. (2009). Silent suffering: Understanding and treating children with selective mutism. *Expert Review of Neurotherapeutics, 9*, 235–243.

Manassis, K., & Levac, A. M. (2004). *Helping your teenager beat depression*. New York: Woodbine House.

Manassis, K., Wilansky-Traynor, P., Farzan, N., Kleiman, V., Parker, K., & Sanford, M. (2010). The Feelings Club: A randomized controlled trial of school-based intervention for anxious and depressed children. *Depression and Anxiety, 27*, 945–952.

March, J. S., Swanson, J. M., Arnold, L. E., Hoza, B., Conners, C. K., Hinshaw, S. P., et al. (2000). Anxiety as a predictor and outcome variable in the Multimodal Treatment Study of Children with ADHD (MTA). *Journal of Abnormal Child Psychology, 28*, 527–541.

Maslow, A. (1954). *Motivation and personality*. New York: Harper & Row.

Mendlowitz, S., Manassis, K., Bradley, S., Scapillato, D., Miezitis, S., & Shaw, B. (1999). Cognitive behavioral group treatments in childhood anxiety disorders: The role of parental involvement. *Journal of the American Academy of Child and Adolescent Psychiatry, 38*, 1223–1229.

Michelson, L., Mannarino, A. P., Marchione, K. E., Stern, M., Figueroa, J., & Beck, S. (1983). A comparative outcome study of behavioral social skills training, interpersonal problem-solving and non-directive control treatments with child psychiatric outpatients. *Behaviour Research and Therapy, 21*(5), 545–556.

Miller, W. R., & Rollnick, S. (2002). *Motivational interviewing: Preparing people for change* (2nd ed.). New York: Guilford Press.

Muato, Z., & Adainez, A. (2005). Does quantity generate quality?: Testing the fundamental principle of brainstorming. *Spanish Journal of Psychology, 8*(2), 215–220.

Mufson, L. (2009). Group interpersonal therapy reduces depression in adolescent survivors of war. *Archives of Disease in Childhood: Education and Practice Edition, 94*(2), 62.

Noam, G. G., & Hermann, C. A. (2002). Where education and mental health meet: Developmental prevention and early intervention in schools. *Development and Psychopathology, 14*(4), 861–875.

Nock, M. K., & Mendes, W. B. (2008). Physiological arousal, distress tolerance, and social problem-solving among adolescent self-injurers. *Journal of Consulting and Clinical Psychology, 76*(1), 28–38.

Nolen-Hoeksema, S., Girgus, J. S., & Seligman, M. E. (1986). Learned helplessness in children: A longitudinal study of depression, achievement, and explanatory style. *Journal of Personality and Social Psychology, 51*, 435–442.

O'Brien, M. P., Zinberg, J. L., Ho, L., Rudd, A., Kopelowicz, A., Daley, M., et al. (2009). Family problem solving interactions and 6-month symptomatic and functional outcomes in youth at ultra-high risk for psychosis and with recent onset psychotic symptoms: A longitudinal study. *Schizophrenia Research, 107*(2–3), 198–205.

Ogrodniczuk, J. S., Joyce, A. S., & Piper, W. E. (2009). Development of the Readiness for Psychotherapy Index. *Journal of Nervous and Mental Disease, 197*(6), 427–433.

Paris, J. (2010). Effectiveness of different psychotherapy approaches in the treatment of borderline personality disorder. *Current Psychiatry Reports, 12,* 56–60.

Park, H. S., & Gaylord-Ross, R. (1989). A problem-solving approach to social skills training in employment settings with mentally retarded youth. *Journal of Applied Behavior Analysis, 22*(4), 373–380.

Phelan, T. W. (2003). *1-2-3 magic: Effective discipline for children 2–12.* Chicago: Child Management.

Pierce, D., & Gunn, J. (2007). GPs' use of problem solving therapy for depression: A qualitative study of barriers to and enablers of evidence based care. *BMC Family Practice, 8,* 24.

POTS Team. (2004). Cognitive behavior therapy, sertraline, and their combination for children and adolescents with obsessive–compulsive disorder: The Pediatric OCD Treatment Study (POTS) randomized controlled trial. *Journal of the American Medical Association, 292,* 1969–1976.

Prochaska, J. O., & DiClemente, C. C. (1984). Self change processes, self efficacy and decisional balance across five stages of smoking cessation. *Progress in Clinical Biological Research, 156,* 131–140.

Prochaska, J. O., DiClemente, C. C., & Norcross, J. C. (1992). In search of how people change: Applications to addictive behaviors. *American Psychologist, 47*(9), 1102–1114.

Pulgaron, E. R., Salamon, K. S., Patterson, C. A., & Barakat, L. P. (2010). A problem-solving intervention for children with persistent asthma: A pilot of a randomized trial at a pediatric summer camp. *Journal of Asthma, 47*(9), 1031–1039.

Reinecke, M. A., Curry, J. F., & March, J. S. (2009). Findings from the Treatment for Adolescents with Depression Study (TADS): What have we learned?: What do we need to know? *Journal of Clinical Child and Adolescent Psychology, 38,* 761–767.

Rueter, M. A., & Conger, R. D. (1998). Reciprocal influences between parenting and adolescent problem-solving behavior. *Developmental Psychology, 34*(6), 1470–1482.

Santor, D. A., & Kusumakar, V. (2001). Open trial of interpersonal therapy in adolescents with moderate to severe major depression: Effectiveness of novice IPT therapists. *Journal of the American Academy of Child and Adolescent Psychiatry, 40,* 236–240.

Scapillato, D., & Manassis, K. (2002). Cognitive-behavioral/interpersonal group treatment for anxious adolescents. *Journal of the American Academy of Child and Adolescent Psychiatry, 41,* 739–741.

Schmidt, H. G., Cohen-Schotanus, J., & Arends, L. R. (2009). Impact of prob-
lem-based, active learning on graduation rates for 10 generations of Dutch
medical students. *Medical Education, 43*(3), 211–218.

Schweickhardt, A., Leta, R., & Bauer, J. (2005). Utilization of psychotherapy
depending on treatment motivation during the diagnostic stage assessed in
an outpatient clinic. *Psychotherapy, Psychosomatic Medicine and Psychology, 55*, 378–385.

Sheeber, L., Allen, N., Davis, B., & Sorensen, E. (2000). Regulation of negative affect during mother–child problem-solving interactions: Adolescent
depressive status and family processes. *Journal of Abnormal Child Psychology, 28*(5), 467–479.

Siegel, J. M., Platt, J. J., & Peizer, S. B. (1976). Emotional and social real-life
problem-solving thinking in adolescent psychiatric patients. *Journal of
Clinical Psychology, 32*(2), 230–232.

Spence, S. H., Sheffield, J. K., & Donovan, C. L. (2003). Preventing adolescent
depression: An evaluation of the Problem Solving for Life program. *Journal of Consulting and Clinical Psychology, 71*(1), 3–13.

Stark, K. D., Reynolds, W. M., & Kaslow, N. J. (1987). A comparison of the
relative efficacy of self-control therapy and a problem-solving therapy for
depression in children. *Journal of Abnormal Child Psychology, 15*(1),
91–113.

Svenson, O., & Jakobsson, M. (2010). Creating coherence in real-life decision
processes: Reasons, differentiation and consolidation. *Scandinavian Journal of Psychology, 51*, 93–102.

Tolstoy, L. (1977). *Anna Karenina.* New York: Macmillan. (Original work published 1877)

Tsukamoto, K., & Sakamoto, A. (2001). The productivity of electronic brainstorming: A comparison of three systems with a control. *Shinrigaku Ken-
kyu, 72*(1), 19–28.

Tulving, E. (2002). Episodic memory: From mind to brain. *Annual Review of
Psychology, 53*, 1–25.

Wade, S. L., Walz, N. C., Carey, J. C., & Williams, K. M. (2008). Prelimi-
nary efficacy of a Web-based family problem-solving treatment program
for adolescents with traumatic brain injury. *Journal of Head Trauma and
Rehabilitation, 23*(6), 369–377.

Wainwright, S. F., Shepard, K. F., Harman, L. B., & Stephens, J. (2010). Novice and experienced physical therapist clinicians: A comparison of how
reflection is used to inform the clinical decision-making process. *Physical
Therapy, 90*, 75–88.

Walkup, J. T., Albano, A. M., Piacentini, J., Birmaher, B., Compton, S. N.,
Sherrill, J., et al. (2008). Cognitive behavioral therapy, sertraline, or a
combination in childhood anxiety. *New England Journal of Medicine,
359*(26), 2753–2766.

Watanabe, K. (2009). Factors behind action, emotion, and decision making.
Brain and Nerve, 61, 1413–1418.

Wearden, A. J., Tarrier, N., Barrowclough, C., Zastowny, T. R., & Rahill, A. A.

(2000). A review of expressed emotion research in health care. *Clinical Psychology Review, 20,* 633–666.

Webster-Stratton, C., Reid, M. J., & Hammond, M. (2004). Treating children with early-onset conduct problems: Intervention outcomes for parent, child, and teacher training. *Journal of Clinical Child and Adolescent Psychology, 33,* 105–124.

Wilson, K. G., Stelzer, J., Bergman, J. N., Kral, M. J., Inayatullah, M., & Elliott, C. A. (1995). Problem solving, stress, and coping in adolescent suicide attempts. *Suicide and Life-Threatening Behavior, 25*(2), 241–252.

Woolgar, M., & Scott, S. (2005). Evidence-based management of conduct disorders. *Current Opinion in Psychiatry, 18,* 392–396.

Yarkoni, T., Braver, T. S., Gray, J. R., & Green, L. (2005). Prefrontal brain activity predicts temporally extended decision-making behavior. *Journal of the Experimental Analysis of Behavior, 84,* 537–554.

Index

f following a page number indicates a figure; *t* following a page number indicates a table.